THE WORDS THEY NEED

THE WORDS THEY NEED

Welcoming Children

Who Are Deaf and Hard of Hearing

To Literacy

Jessica Stelling

The book was manufactured in the United States of America.
Typography by The Type Shoppe, Inc.
Printing and binding by McNaughton & Gunn.
Cover Design by Jean Brunel.

ISBN 0-912752-44-0

Library of Congress Cataloging-in-Publication Data
Stelling, Jessica, 1942–
    The words they need : welcoming children who are deaf and
    hard of hearing to literacy / Jessica Stelling.
        p.   cm.
    Includes bibliographical references and index.
    ISBN 0-912752-44-0 (pbk.)
    1. Deaf—Education—Reading.   2. Reading (Elementary)
    3. Language arts (Elementary) I. Title.
    HV2469.R4S74 1997   97-29493
    371.91'2—dc21   CIP

Contents

To children who walk a long road to language learning.
To all their teachers.

Preface

As a teacher, I have mentors whom I have never met.

My first acquaintance with deafness came from a magazine article about Helen Keller and Anne Sullivan. Their story moved me powerfully, even at age eight. Soon afterward, *The Miracle Worker* made its own indelible impression. Much later, Anne Sullivan's words would speak to me as one teacher to another. But nothing has exceeded the impact of those original encounters.

Early in my teaching experience, I became acquainted with the work of New Zealand educator Sylvia Ashton-Warner. Ashton-Warner dedicated herself to helping young Maori children make the transition from nonreading to reading. The children's cultural background was not reflected in the standard European primers. Instead, Ashton-Warner used the children's own language to start them on the road to reading and writing. The idea of using children's own words as the basis for developing language spoke to me at a time when I had not yet gained competence and confidence as a teacher. In Ashton-Warner's work, I found a vision of the teacher I wished to be.

Ashton-Warner was an exponent of integrated language learning at a time when this was not common educational practice. Decades later, whole language evolved as a reaction to rote, fragmented language learning. Whole language engages children in a process in which reading and writing develop hand in hand, one reinforcing the other. By the time whole language had gained widespread acceptance, my work with children had already taken shape in that direction. The ideas and spirit of the whole language movement have helped me bring children with hearing impairments closer to loving language and using it well.

For nearly two decades, the Writing Project of Columbia University Teachers College (Calkins with Harwayne 1991) has been a vibrant example of integrated language learning in action. Reading, writing, and language are closely intertwined as teachers and children explore the process of writing. In example after example, Writing Project teachers convey the breadth and depth of young children's grasp of all aspects of the creative writing process. Some of these abilities are beyond the reach of many school-age deaf and hard-of-hearing children, who are still developing and consolidating basic language. Even so, what is possible for some children has opened my eyes to possibilities for hearing-impaired children as well.

The language experience approach, including aspects of the Writing Project, underlies the teaching and learning described in this book. At the same time, a structured approach to phonics has come to children's aid as a tool for reading and writing words that are not in their sight vocabulary. This aspect of reading is derived from, and subordinate to, reading for meaning and content. Integrating a multisensory approach to phonics in a natural language program has enabled some children to partake more fully of all that whole language has to offer.

The Words They Need has grown out of my work with children who are mainstreamed in regular classes. The book reflects specific aspects of my teaching experience. First, it describes children who have entered school at a lower level of language development than is characteristic of many mainstreamed children or many children in self-contained programs. Second, it is based on my work in an oral setting.

A range of possibilities pertaining to modes of communication and educational settings is open to families of children who are deaf or hard of hearing. Children brought up orally are exposed to spoken language from the beginning; those who grow up with American Sign Language have ASL as their native language.

Like every language, ASL is complete in itself and expressive in its own unique way. Information, thoughts, and feelings are communicated as effectively through ASL as through any other language. The words of ASL, no less than those of spoken English, bring children "life and growth and refreshment." But because ASL has no written counterpart, it is essential that school-age children become literate in English as well.

In discussing children's needs and how to meet them, I have at times made reference to verbal shortcomings, language deficits, and dearth of language experience. These observations point to the limited exposure to language in the early lives of the children on whom this book is based. These same observations do not apply to children entering school with more highly developed oral language. Neither do they apply to children with a solid knowledge of ASL, whose need is to bring their language mastery to bear on the acquisition of English as a second language.

Throughout this book, the word "language" refers specifically to the development of skills leading to literacy in English. This is not at odds with an appreciation of ASL as a valid communicative and educational choice. Educators of children who are deaf and hard of hearing share common ground in their commitment to children's acquiring a high level of proficiency in English. It is this educational process that is addressed in *The Words They Need*. My hope is that the book will be of value to parents and teachers in helping children develop English language competence, whatever their communicative preference.

Insight into the needs of children who are deaf and hard of hearing may shed light on the needs of children who struggle with language for other reasons as well. All children with language delays and/or impairments benefit from systematic exposure to language—both spontaneous and carefully guided—as they develop the vocabulary, sentence structure, and abstract thinking abilities that come naturally to others. It is for these children, and for all who join in bringing them the gifts of language and literacy, that this book has been written.

In writing *The Words They Need*, I have been deeply influenced by educators whose work has struck a chord in me, and is inextricably woven into my own. In the same way, I invite you to gravitate toward those ideas and approaches that feel natural and enjoyable to you, and to adapt or disregard others that seem alien in some way.

Jessica Stelling
1997

Acknowledgments

The Words They Need owes its origins to an independent study sabbatical granted by the New York City Board of Education. Colleagues in various disciplines have helped give shape to this writing. The feedback of Sue Behn, Dan Bergman, Gloria Duffy, Lucille Duncan, Rosemarie Kolb, Hindy List, Tom Olsen, Blanche Saia, and Elizabeth Scully encouraged me to persevere beyond the early stages of writing. Around that time, Shelley Harwayne's enthusiasm for the anecdotal material strongly influenced the direction and, ultimately, the nature of the book.

This project has been enriched by the collective knowledge and expertise of Anise Baron, Terry Coyle, Richard Duncan, Annette Elias, Howard Fink, Ruth Green, Judith Kaplan, Annette Lust, Karin Mango, Chani Monoker, Sheila Rabin, and Mary Rowe. Each one has been available for consultation on an array of issues throughout the course of this undertaking.

The insightful reading of Elizabeth Ying and Patricia Rothschild helped refine the manuscript as it neared completion.

For more than two decades, the League for the Hard of Hearing has contributed to my understanding of the educational needs of children with hearing impairments. The staff of the League responded generously and immediately to a variety of needs that arose during the writing of this book.

The cover of *The Words They Need* was inspired by Virginia Roberts and created as a labor of love by Jean Brunel.

Every stage and aspect of *The Words They Need*, from its inception through the moment of publication, has been touched by the collaboration of Darlynne Devenny. Darlynne's sharing of her knowledge and experience has been the highest expression of what one friend and colleague can do for another.

The staff and affiliates of York Press have carefully shepherded *The Words They Need* through the many processes involved in preparing a manuscript for publication. Working with Elinor Hartwig has been a true collaboration enhanced by mutual respect and many moments of shared laughter. Our partnership has made this one of the most satisfying and pleasurable stages in the life of the book.

I have learned how many people it takes to create a book. Each of them has, in the words of Robert Louis Stevenson, given the manuscript "a just and patient hearing." Each has my deepest gratitude for his or her gifts of time, warmth, humor, and professional understanding. Each has become an integral part of *The Words They Need*.

Permissions

We thank all those who have given permission to reprint material in this book. We have made every effort to acquire permission from copyright holders. We regret any oversights and will gladly correct the problem in future printings.

Excerpt from *Educational Care*, by Melvin Levine. Copyright 1994 by Melvin Levine. Reprinted with kind permission of Educators Publishing Service.

Excerpt from *Children of Silence: The Story of My Daughter's Triumph Over Deafness*, by Kathy Robinson. Copyright 1987 © 1990 by Kathy Robinson. Originally published (1987) by Victor Gollancz Ltd. Used by permission of Dutton Signet, a division of Penguin Books USA, Inc., and of The Carol Smith Literary Agency.

Excerpts from *Assessment and Management of Mainstreamed Hearing-Impaired Children*, by Mark Ross, Diane Brackett, and Antonia Brancia Maxon. Copyright 1991 by PRO-ED, Inc. Reprinted with permission.

Excerpt from "Helping Your Child Succeed in School," by Katherine Foran and David Heim. © 1994 in *Adoptive Parents* (September-October). Used with permission.

Excerpts from *Hearing Impairments in Young Children*, by Arthur Boothroyd. © 1982 by Prentice-Hall, Inc. and 1988 by Alexander Graham Bell Association for the Deaf. Used with permission.

Excerpts from "Essentials of a Communication Curriculum" by Michael Breene and Christopher Candlin. In *Applied Linguistics*, 1,2, Summer, 1980. Used by permission of Oxford University Press.

Excerpt from "A Graduate Speaks" by Alexis Patrizio. In *The Listening Post* (Spring):4–5. Used with permission of The Helen Beebe Center.

Excerpts from *Child's Talk: Learning to Use Language*, by Jerome Bruner. © 1983 by W. W. Norton and Company and by Oxford University Press. Reprinted by permission of W. W. Norton & Company, Inc., and of Oxford University Press.

Quotation from *Daybook: Journal of an Artist* by Ann Truitt. Pantheon Books, New York. Copyright © 1984 by Ann Truitt. Reprinted by permission of author. All rights reserved.

Introduction

Levine (1994) speaks of the compassionate meeting of children's individual needs as "educational care." *The Words They Need* is concerned with the educational care of children with developmental needs in all aspects of language. This book was written for teachers, parents, and clinicians who work to overcome the language delays that prevent children from participating in life to the fullest extent possible.

Hearing children achieve language mastery long before school age. Children who are deaf and hard of hearing require systematic language development in order to acquire basic vocabulary, grammar, syntax, and general information. Learning to read and write is an overwhelming task for hearing-impaired children who enter school with significant deficits in these areas.

The Words They Need has evolved from my experiences with deaf and hard-of-hearing children in a public elementary school. These children have received resource room support while attending general education classes. The book examines the teaching and learning of language in the resource room setting.

STRUCTURE OF THE BOOK

The first four chapters identify needs associated with hearing impairment and provide basic information related to hearing loss, audiological testing, and amplification devices. These chapters describe the role of the resource room teacher, and introduce three of the seventeen children whose progress unfolds throughout the book.

Chapters 5–18 address the remediation of deficits and the development of basic skills in language, reading, and writing.

Chapters 19–22 describe children whose difficulties are greater than those typically encountered in the resource room setting. This section reflects on achieving a balance between the efficiency of a clinical session and the leisure essential to growth and learning. It examines the concept of inclusion as it applies to the needs of hearing-impaired children attending regular classes with resource room support.

Chapters 23–25 examine children's language needs from the perspective of nine educational researchers. This section discusses the interplay between "relevance" and self-esteem. It reflects on ways in which we, as teachers, can give ourselves what we need in order to sustain the difficult effort of offering children the best of our knowledge, experience, and judgment.

Appendix A provides a glossary of terms. Appendix B gives auditory and language profiles of the children who appear throughout the book. A small number of children are presented only once or twice in the course of the book. Others appear and reappear in different contexts. In several instances, it is possible to follow the children's progress in a variety of areas. The Profiles of Children provide a basis for understanding children's strengths and needs. While the children's names have been changed, all learning experiences took place as described.

The Words They Need embodies a natural language philosophy that invites teachers to let their work be shaped by the needs and experiences of their children. Throughout the book, natural language learning is depicted side by side with more obviously structured, teacher-directed activities. At times, the teacher's guiding hand is subtle in providing a format that supports learning or gives shape to a child's response. Such moments have the feeling of natural language learning.

At other times, obstacles to learning need to be removed with the help of prescriptive activities that are not only structured but also initiated by the teacher. These situations, which may appear to be at odds with whole language learning, provide the foundation from which more spontaneous learning can proceed. Once mastered, activities initiated and/or structured by the teacher are restored to context, there to become integrated into each child's fund of information and knowledge.

The Words They Need includes reading, writing, and language activities that have been helpful to particular children. When adapting other teachers' ideas, it is imperative to shape and reshape them to the current child's level, situation, and learning style. Without the perceptive matching of our teaching approaches to students' learning needs, the most promising activity is at risk of becoming rigid and losing much of its value.

The natural or integrated approach to language learning is rooted in this responsiveness to children's needs, which evolves by means of constant evaluation and reevaluation. In this process, intellect and intuition combine to create teaching that is flexible and dynamic. There are no all-purpose solutions to the challenges inherent in teaching and learning. A method in which every step is specified contradicts the essence of natural language learning. In keeping with this philosophy, activities described throughout the book are offered as raw material, to be adapted and adjusted as needed.

In her keynote speech at a Teachers College Writing Project Conference, Newbery award-winner Katherine Paterson spoke passionately about the need for children's literature. Paterson voiced her conviction that "to give the children of the world **the words they need** is to give them life and growth and refreshment."

These words, which still ring in my ears, express better than any others my wish for children who are deaf and hard of hearing.

Chapter 1

"Once Upon a Time . . ."

PETER PAN: A MOTHER'S JOURNEY

"Once upon a time there were three children who lived in London . . ."

My spirits plunged. How could I tell Sarah the story of Peter Pan when she couldn't even understand the first sentence? . . . Sarah was starting school in four months. Time was running out.

I decided that as Sarah and Joanne knew what "children" meant, I would start with "three." "Count my fingers," I said. "One, two, three. Here are three buttons. Count them with me. One . . ."

"Waa." Sarah held up one finger.

"Do." Joanne held up four fingers, then covered two with her other hand.

"Three," I said . . .

I went to the window. "Look. Can you see the birds in the trees?" They came to look and I said, "Birds live in trees. Where does Mandy live?" I pointed to her house. "Mandy lives there. She lives in a house."

We followed this with picture cards. We put the snail in its shell and the bee in the hive. "The snail lives in his shell. The bee lives in a hive," I told them and we all trooped outside to look for a snail.

It rained in the afternoon but this didn't stop us going in search of a "village." I had drawn pictures of a village before we left and there was an anticipatory air in the car as Sarah and Joanne competed to be the first to spot one.

1

"Dere," Joanne shouted, as she pointed to the tops of houses showing above the trees.

A village however is smaller than a town. A town has more shops and offices. We went to our nearest town.

But a town isn't as big as a city. A city had a cathedral, and many more shops, offices, houses and factories. We went to stay with Jimmy and Barbara, friends of ours, who lived in a city called London. . . .

I felt excessively pleased with myself. It had taken eight weeks and we had got as far as, "There were three children who lived in London." All I had to do now was to give Sarah the idea of "Once upon a time. . . ."

One memorable day I lifted Sarah and Joanne on to the settee and opened the book of Peter Pan again. "Listen to this story," I said.

"Once upon a time there were three children who lived in London. Their names were Wendy, Michael and John. They lived in an enormous house with an attic, a room under the roof. Their parents were called Mr and Mrs Darling. Daddy and I are called Mr and Mrs Robinson. They had a dog called Nana, and she was a special dog. There weren't many dogs like her; she did special things. She looked after the children and gave them a spoonful of medicine every single night—Monday, Tuesday . . ."

"Uggh." Sarah pulled a face when I showed her the picture. "I doh li mediee."

"The children all loved Nana but she was very strict."

Joanne copied my frown.

"One night when it was extremely dark—very, very dark—a boy called Peter Pan came to London. Peter Pan was an orphan, he had no Mummy or Daddy. He fell out of his pram when he was a baby."

Sarah's eyes were as wide as saucers, and Joanne looked as if she was trying to work this out in her head.

"Peter Pan could fly, and he flew to London to find his shadow. He had lost it."

I got up and stood in front of the window so that my shadow fell across the floor. "His shadow."

"I do id doo." Joanne scrambled down from the settee, falling on the floor in her haste.

Shadows take time *and it was another ten minutes before we sat down again.*

"When he got to the house someone barked loudly . . ."

"Gaga."

"Yes it was Nana . . . What a lovely *story this is"*

(Robinson 1987, 90–94).

Step by step, this energetic and creative mother brings a beloved childhood story within reach of her two little girls, both profoundly deaf. When Kathy Robinson first sat down with four-year-old Sarah and two-year-old Joanne and began to read to them, lack of language rendered the words meaningless. Unable to comprehend the story, the girls wriggled off her lap before the end of the first sentence.

More than two months elapsed. During that time, Mrs. Robinson found ways to translate every detail from the opening lines of the book into a concrete learning experience with language attached. One unforgettable day, the three of them gathered to attempt again the story of Peter Pan. This time the children listened with rapt attention, caught up in the story line.

Kathy Robinson's work contains the quintessential elements of helping young deaf and hard-of-hearing children acquire language. Experience, language, and reading blend into a seamless whole. Stumbling blocks are excerpted, clarified, and restored to context.

What this mother accomplished with her two preschool children stands as a model of what is possible given an abundance of time and individual attention. *The Words They Need* examines teaching methods and philosophies that come to our aid as we work toward language development in the more restricted school setting.

Chapter 2

The Resource Room Setting

Two hard-of-hearing children entered kindergarten at the same time. Dominique had a mild hearing loss compounded by extreme difficulty focusing her attention in a listening situation. Crystal had a severe hearing loss and little auditory training before entering the mainstreamed setting. (See Appendix B for speech, hearing, and language profiles of individual children.)

Dominique, whose learning needs are described more fully in Chapter 19, was a reticent child who answered monosyllabically and seldom volunteered any spontaneous conversation. Crystal was highly verbal but had, at most, a few hundred words at her command.

As we walked down the hall to the resource room, I looked for things to comment on: Crystal's haircut, Dominique's new shoes. Dominique was likely to offer one-word answers, and occasionally could be coaxed into volunteering a bit more, while Crystal was eager to elaborate to the best of her ability. One or another of the girls' comments usually lent itself to being expanded into a structured conversation.

Ms. S.:	Crystal, remember what you told us about your tooth when we were coming down the stairs?
Crystal:	My tooth fell out.
Ms. S.:	Dominique, what did Crystal say?
Dominique:	I don't know.
Ms. S.:	Ask her.
Dominique:	What did you say, Crystal?

Dominique's distractibility interfered with accurate listening and appropriate responses. It was necessary to focus and refocus her attention on the person speaking. Several repetitions were often required before she was able to demonstrate her awareness of what was being discussed by repeating or rephrasing what Crystal had volunteered.

Crystal did not share Dominique's difficulty attending to the speaker. Rather, the severity of her hearing loss made listening a challenge for her. Discussions sparked by the girls' experiences provided a context for sharpening and refining Crystal's emerging auditory skills.

These structured exchanges, at first more stilted than spontaneous, remained a major resource room activity for two-and-one-half years. As time went on, listening and responding became easier and more natural for both girls. The need for guided discussions gradually diminished, as conversational skills became incorporated into other activities.

DESCRIPTION OF PROGRAM

The resource room depicted in *The Words They Need* is a pull-out program specifically for children who are deaf and hard of hearing. Children spend their days in regular education classes. They are assigned to the resource room by the Committee on Special Education. Placement is determined by a battery of speech, language, educational, and psychological assessments. The resulting IEPs (Individualized Educational Plans) of children such as Crystal and Dominique indicate the need for a daily 45-minute period of resource room support. For these children, self-contained programs with the option of selective mainstreaming have been ruled out in favor of full-time placement in regular education classes.

The evaluation and placement process is a legally mandated outgrowth of Public Law 94-142, the Individuals with Disabilities Education Act (Code of Federal Regulations 1993). This law came into being to ensure that every child with special needs receive a free, appropriate public education.

In the resource room, children learn to comprehend language using speechreading (lipreading) coupled with auditory training to the maximum extent possible. These, together with the development of grammar, syntax, and vocabulary, form the core of resource room work. The structure of the curriculum and the manner in which these areas are introduced and developed are determined by the individual resource room teacher.

Reading and writing are affected by language delays. At the same time, both are avenues to language acquisition. This gives them an important place in resource room programming.

A Team Effort

The nature and level of work undertaken in the resource room depends, in part, on the extent of the child's learning before he or she enters school. Some beginning resource room children are farther along than others in their language development. Older children entering the resource room program for the first time may exhibit delays nearly as great as those of younger ones. Early amplification, combined with a foundation in language and literacy, are essential if deaf and hard-of-hearing children are to take their place as active participants in the mainstreamed setting early in their school lives.

Effective mainstreaming requires a cooperative effort between classroom teacher, resource room teacher, parents, and child. With this teamwork in place, it is realistic for classroom teachers to extend their expectations for the class to the deaf or hard-of-hearing child, with appropriate modifications. For guidelines for classroom teachers of mainstreamed hearing-impaired children, see Ross et al. (1991).

Resource room teachers, for their part, make the work of the class accessible to the child, while continuously reinforcing and expanding language concepts. Parents, under the guidance of speech and language clinicians, provide academic support on a daily basis, while furthering the child's language development informally throughout the day. Children contribute to their own success by a combination of self-motivation and openness to being taught.

CRITERIA FOR SUCCESSFUL MAINSTREAMING

A child's skills and potential are important factors in considering appropriate class placement. Ross et al. (1991) suggest criteria that make mainstreaming feasible. In order to benefit from a general education setting, a child needs to:

- have age-appropriate classroom, social, and interactive behaviors;
- fit into an established group in the selected class with respect to language and academic performance;

- coordinate maximal use of auditory cues with visual cues via hearing aids and FM units;

- speak intelligibly to teachers and classmates;

- have the receptive language required to comprehend classroom material and conversational exchanges;

- have the expressive language required to participate in class discussions and to communicate with teachers and classmates;

- integrate socially into a peer group;

- assume some responsibility for his or her own education; and

- be adaptable and capable of handling changes in routines (p. 73).

Birch (1975) suggests that superior reading and receptive skills may compensate for lower expressive skills, and vice versa. He proposes that being integrated in regular class activities may in itself lead to improvement in communication skills.

A MAINSTREAMING MODEL

"Why did Robin Hood and his men believe that they could not expect to receive justice at the hands of the Sheriff of Nottingham?" Using this question from a hypothetical lesson plan of a fourth- or fifth-grade teacher, Birch outlines a three-part strategy for making grade-level work accessible to the mainstreamed hearing-impaired child.

- Lesson material is shared in routine conferences between classroom and resource room teachers. The resource room teacher then *preteaches* the topic in a twenty-minute session prior to the regular class. An abstract concept such as "justice" or an idiomatic expression such as "at the hands of . . ." may call for clarification. Preteaching is concluded when the resource room teacher is satisfied that the child is ready to enter into the regular teacher's instructional period on equal terms with his or her hearing classmates.

- The classroom teacher *teaches* the lesson and reports any problems encountered by the deaf or hard-of-hearing child.

- In a *postteaching* session, the resource room teacher fills in gaps related to language, preparation, or background.

As children gain in knowledge and skills, they are expected to assume a greater share of responsibility for their own schoolwork. They learn to take the initiative in asking for assistance. At the same time, children are discouraged from seeking help with work they are capable of undertaking on their own. As children become independent learners, the preteach-teach-postteach pattern phases itself out.

A Different Situation

The preteach-teach-postteach model takes for granted that children are adequately prepared for full class participation at their grade level. The situation is different for children with significant language deficits. In the absence of early intervention, language development replaces academic support as the primary focus of the resource room teacher. It becomes his or her task to lay a foundation in word knowledge, sentence and question formation, and the give and take of basic conversation. Sentence length and complexity need to be expanded as the child's language grows. Synonyms, antonyms, idioms, grammatical and syntactical structures, and abstract thinking abilities need to be introduced and brought to higher and higher levels.

For many reasons, it has been difficult for most families of the children in this book to meet their youngsters' language and learning needs. As a result, these children typically manifest significant deficits at the most basic levels of language, reading, writing, and general knowledge. At age five or six, children can probably name at least a number of common everyday objects. They may be able to answer *who* and *what* questions. They may recognize cat and elephant, table and chair, without necessarily being able to categorize them as animals or furniture. In order for children to follow a story line, it may be necessary to reduce the story to its most concrete essentials, relate it in familiar vocabulary, and provide additional clarification by drawing or acting it out. Having experienced the story, children may be virtually unable to retell it without a great deal of repetition and assistance.

Young resource room children may not be able to count to ten or recite the alphabet. They may not be familiar with days of the week and months of the year. *Yesterday, today,* and *tomorrow* may or may not have meaning for them. They may or may not be able to relate home or school happenings in a comprehensible way. They may express themselves telegraphically: "Daddy-Jimmy-go-store-two-car-pow."

Like all children, children who are deaf and hard of hearing are most likely to comprehend and use frequently encountered words and phrases: "Come here." "Where's Mommy?" "Time for lunch." Like all children, they gain language related to individual experiences. What is missing is the broad language base that most children acquire without being specifically taught.

Hearing children gain this foundation by absorbing language that goes on around them, along with language directed at them. This happens with a minimum of conscious effort on the part of the adults in their environment. In contrast, hearing-impaired children in the early stages of language development need to have their attention deliberately focused on each new word. Consequently, a young deaf or hard-of-hearing child may walk down a city street pointing out gargoyles, without yet being able to name or identify more basic words such as *fork* or *spoon*.

The adoptive parents of two school-age children from South America describe how "helping Anna and Carlos catch up and keep up was like starting to build the Empire State Building on the twentieth floor. For every floor we added to the top, we had to add to the bottom" (Foran and Heim 1994, 24). Their description pinpoints the educational challenge facing parents and teachers of hearing-impaired children.

The discrepancy between higher level learning and basic deficits is prolonged when school provides the child's only language and academic support. Eight-year-old Douglas poses searching questions about the life of Dr. Martin Luther King, Jr. Yet when asked which word does not belong, he reasons that blue does not belong with yellow, brown, and seven because "it's another color." Douglas' interest and intelligence have catapulted his learning to the "twentieth floor" with regard to his ability to grasp and discuss so profound a subject as civil rights. In comparison, his inability to categorize basic words reflects his uneven language foundation.

A TEACHER'S DILEMMA

The contrast between bursts of age-appropriate learning and weaknesses in fundamental areas poses a dilemma. Both ends of the continuum are essential to children's growth as learners. Limiting instruction to language drills would deprive a child like Douglas of the intellectual stimulation that spurs language development. On the other hand, concentrating exclusively on mind-broadening and emotionally satisfying reading and discussion would ultimately curtail Douglas' understanding and ability to express himself.

In the resource room, pace and language can be adjusted to facilitate comprehension. Missing concepts can be filled in. A simple allusion to previously learned material may be all that is needed to prepare Douglas for the topic at hand. Douglas' understanding and ability to express his thoughts reflect the individualized attention available to him in this setting. These same strengths are little in evidence in the classroom, where the individualization he continues to need is seldom possible.

TWO CHILDREN

Crystal came to the resource room asking for help with a sixth-grade assignment. She was to read three short stories and describe the mood, plot, and theme of each.

In conveying the mood of de Maupassant's *The Necklace* (1967), Crystal wrote that "the story seems so gloomy and sad because the girl worked like a slave for ten years to cover up a mistake." The plot centers around a selfish girl who "loses a worthless necklace and thinks its [sic] valuable. It belonged to a friend. She depletes her savings and she worked for ten years to buy a diamond necklace that she had misplaced. At the end she discovers that the necklace that she misplaced is worthless." The theme, in Crystal's words, is that of "a woman who thinks it matters what other people say about her being poor and about having to look perfect no matter what."

Because the language of short stories tends to be difficult, I had provided an anthology and suggested two stories I thought Crystal might enjoy. We began each of them together. Crystal finished them at home, along with a third. Crystal's written response was entirely her own. My contribution was to offer the word "depletes," and give her the opportunity to find and correct errors in spelling.

That same month, John's fourth-grade teacher assigned a research project on animals. A set of guidelines explained every step of the report. Children worked independently, in and outside the classroom, consulting with the teacher as needed.

For John, however, this became a resource room undertaking. The first challenge was finding a picture book simple enough for him to participate in reading. Extensive questioning and discussion were required before John could digest and relate the three or four sentences presented on each page. Recording the information was a long and tedious process. The project took four weeks of resource room time. It left John little closer to independence as a reader, writer, or researcher than he had been when we started.

Making a Choice

John and Crystal exemplify two very different situations. By sixth grade, Crystal had begun to approach grade level in the knowledge and skills required for meaningful mainstreaming. At this stage, an increasingly close, cooperative team relationship between classroom and resource room teachers became possible. The preteach-teach-postteach strategy came into play as a way of fostering maximum participation in the regular class setting.

For John, independence was still a distant goal. He lacked the basic skills that would have enabled him to enter into a learning partnership on any aspect of his class project.

In my experience, scrambling to make assignment after assignment accessible to children before they have acquired fundamental skills has not resulted in giving children the foundation they need. Deceptively good work can be accomplished with a disproportionate amount of teacher input. At best, this can give children who are ready, an experience that will enable them to participate more fully in future endeavors. At worst, working consistently above a child's level perpetuates dependence on the resource room teacher without enabling the child to move toward independent learning with an appropriate degree of support.

A profoundly deaf college-bound high school senior expressed her gratitude to the speech and hearing clinic that helped make her social, recreational, and academic achievements possible. The clinic "didn't teach me to do any of these things," explained Patrizio (1995, 5). It was, rather, help in the form of language development and guidance that "allowed me the opportunity to do all of these things."

Similarly, I have found that pursuing a cohesive but separate resource room course of study offers the best opportunity to ground children in the kinds of learning that prepare them for fuller class participation until such time as meaningful integration becomes possible.

SUMMARY

In the absence of early and continuous parental involvement in the language and academic spheres, it takes time for children to develop a foundation in all areas of language and learning. As children move toward grade level in one area or another, it becomes feasible to integrate language development with class activities and projects. Book reports, compositions, science projects, and social studies assignments can all serve as a basis for the application and further development of reading, writing, and language skills. Until then, the resource room remains responsible for both the "top" and the "bottom" of the educational ladder. This is an overwhelming assignment.

Resource room teachers are faced with a two-fold task: to remediate deficits that date back to earliest years, while helping children approach grade level in all school areas. In so doing, the resource room teacher ascertains each child's level and moves on from there. The skill and patience of speech, classroom, and auxiliary teachers, coupled with resource room support, enable children to experience success and satisfaction at every step of the way.

Chapter 3

Understanding Hearing Impairment

TYPES OF HEARING LOSS

Hearing loss may be conductive or sensorineural.

A **conductive loss** is the impeding of sound transmission to the inner ear. Conductive losses typically result from otitis media (middle ear infections), perforation of the tympanic membrane, and/or the accumulation of wax in the external canal. Congenital malformations of the ossicles (bones in the middle ear) also result in moderate to severe losses. Many conductive conditions can be medically or surgically treated, resulting in improved hearing.

A **sensorineural loss** results from damage to the cochlea or auditory nerve. Sensorineural hearing loss is permanent, and is accompanied by a reduction in sound quality and clarity. Most resource room children have sensorineural losses.

A **mixed hearing loss** is a combination of a conductive loss and a sensorineural loss.

For further information regarding all aspects of hearing loss, see Boothroyd (1988, 42–56).

Assessing Hearing Loss

Audiologists generally test hearing by presenting pure tones at octave or semi-octave intervals from 125 to 8000 Herz (frequency expressed in cycles per second). Each ear is tested separately. A threshold for a particular frequency is established by presenting an audible tone, then reducing the intensity until the listener is unable to detect the tone.

Testing is conducted in a soundproof room using a calibrated audiometer. The child is instructed to raise his or her hand upon hearing a tone, and is then fitted with earphones. Young children are tested with play audiometry, in which they drop a toy in a can for each tone heard. This, and similar procedures, are intended simply to help maintain the interest of the child.

Thresholds for pure tones are recorded on an audiogram and are measured in decibels (dB). The testing equipment is calibrated in such a way that 0 dBHL (dB Hearing Level) represents the level at which average young adults without hearing problems can just detect the presence of the pure tone.

Degrees of Hearing Loss

The following information is derived largely from Anderson and Matkin (1991). Two measurements are referred to throughout this section. Herz (Hz) denotes sound frequency, or pitch. Decibels (dB) or decibels Hearing Level (dBHL) refers to volume, or loudness, of a sound.

Hearing is **normal** when the child's responses fall between 0 and 25 dBHL. A child with hearing sensitivity between 0 and 15 dBHL will detect the complete speech signal even at soft conversational levels.

Children whose hearing is **borderline normal** (16 to 25 dBHL) may not hear the rustling of leaves or the chirping of birds. They may miss faint or distant speech. This can occur in a noisy classroom or when the teacher is more than three feet away. Children may be unaware of subtle conversational cues or miss portions of fast-paced peer interactions, causing them to appear awkward or react inappropriately. The listening effort required in the classroom may result in fatigue.

Thresholds in the 25 to 40 dBHL range constitute a **mild** hearing loss. A child with a mild loss may not hear whispering, the ticking of a clock, or voiceless sibilants such as /s/, /f/, and /th/. Without amplification, a child with a 35 dB loss may miss at least 50% of class discussions. Children with mild losses are thought to be daydreaming, hearing when they want to, or not paying attention. The term "mild" is misleading in view of the impact this degree of hearing loss can have on language comprehension, expression, and the articulation of high frequency speech sounds.

A **moderate** hearing loss falls between 40 and 55 dBHL. A child with a moderate loss is likely to have a mild articulation problem. Without amplification, a child with a 40 dB loss may miss 50% to 75% of the speech signal; a child with a 50 dB loss may miss 80% to 100%. Children with hearing loss in the moderate range are likely to have delayed or defective syntax, limited vocabulary, and mild articulation problems. Communication is often significantly affected; socialization with peers becomes increasingly difficult.

A 55 to 70 dBHL loss is considered to be **moderate-severe**. Without amplification, conversation must be very loud to be understood. Children have very reduced vocabularies and multiple misarticulations of consonants. They are likely to have delayed language and syntax and reduced speech intelligibility. Children may require special help in all language skills and language-based academic subjects, as well as with reading and writing.

A **severe** hearing loss lies in the 70 to 90 dBHL range. The term "hard of hearing" still applies. Without amplification, a child with a severe hearing loss can identify some environmental sounds, hear loud voices close to the ear, and discriminate vowels but not all consonants. Speech and language are both severely impaired. With amplification, a child should be able to identify environmental sounds and detect all the sounds of speech.

Children who do not hear sound until it is at least 90 dBHL have a **profound** hearing loss. Some children may be unable to hear at some frequencies regardless of volume. Voice production is aberrant, with little variation in intonation. Children with severe and profound hearing losses do not develop speech and language without intensive intervention.

Children with a **unilateral** loss (normal hearing in one ear and at least a mild, permanent loss in the other) have difficulty localizing sounds and voices. They may have difficulty hearing faint or distant speech. They will have greater difficulty understanding speech when the environment is noisy or reverberant. These children have difficulty detecting or understanding soft speech coming from the side of the bad ear, especially during group discussions. They may appear inattentive or frustrated.

The most common cause of **fluctuating** hearing loss is recurrent ear infections. Because hearing is unreliable and unpredictable, children "do not integrate sound adequately into their general perceptual development and they do not give sound the priority it deserves" (Boothroyd 1988, 55). Reduced auditory attention frequently results in delayed speech and language development, as well as in problems with auditory processing and memory. Hearing loss resulting from otitis media during the early, critical years of language acquisition may have long-term auditory consequences.

A TYPICAL HEARING LOSS

A hearing loss may not be the same at every frequency. For children with sensorineural hearing losses, hearing is often better in the low frequencies and poorer in the high frequencies. This gives the audiogram a slope.

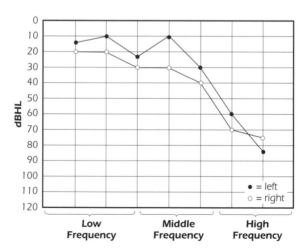

Children with this type of hearing loss can detect the presence of sound with relative ease, yet have difficulty differentiating sounds. This is a particular problem for understanding speech. Children appear to respond inconsistently when the low frequencies they hear best are masked by environmental noise. Children may be able to hear the voice of the speaker and, perhaps, distinguish vowel sounds, yet be unable to hear consonant sounds. Unless amplification is carefully chosen for these children, the amplified low-frequency speech sounds they hear may mask the consonant sounds, which lie predominantly in the high frequencies.

A hearing loss may not be symmetrical (similar in both ears). Children with a large discrepancy in hearing sensitivity between ears will have difficulty hearing sound coming from the direction of the poorer ear. They will also have difficulty localizing the direction of the source of sound, since localizing requires binaural hearing.

The children described throughout this book represent a range of hearing losses. In addition, children bring with them their own histories. This combination of factors is reflected in each child's constellation of strengths and weaknesses.

HEARING AID EVALUATION

In order to determine the effectiveness of amplification, children are tested with their hearing aids in a soundproof room. First, the audiologist determines the Speech Reception Threshold or SRT (level at which a child correctly repeats 50% of a spondee word list. Spondee words are equally accented compound words such as *mailman, baseball,* and *hotdog*). Volume settings on the hearing aids are chosen to give an SRT as close to the normal range (0-25 dBHL) as possible. Second, speech discrimination is tested at normal conversational level (50 dBHL) and at quiet conversational level (35 dBHL). Third, the child's tolerance for amplification is checked by gradually increasing the loudness of the sound until the child shows signs of discomfort.

Inserting a computerized probe microphone directly into the child's ear canal while the hearing aid is in place makes it possible to assess objectively how the child perceives sound. Probe microphone measurement, or Real Ear Testing, allows the examiner to determine how sound is being modified by the child's hearing aid, earmold, and ear canal resonance. Real Ear

Testing supplements subjective methods of hearing aid selection and assessment. For further information, see Mueller (1992).

FM Units

Hearing aids provide optimum benefit when the child is within three feet of the speaker and there is little or no background noise. This situation seldom prevails in the classroom. Teachers need to circulate around the room; the sounds of voices, movement, pencils, and paper cannot be eliminated. Because hearing aids amplify all sounds equally, it is difficult for children with reduced hearing to identify and attend to the speaker's voice in the presence of competing background noise.

Amplification devices called FM units reduce the negative effect of distance and background noise. Each child's unit is paired with a teacher microphone. Just as FM radios receive transmissions from a broadcasting station, the FM unit picks up the teacher's voice, which is forwarded to the child's own hearing aids. As a result, the teacher's voice retains the same strength and clarity no matter where he or she is in the room or even beyond. A switch gives the child the option of focusing on the teacher, or letting in a broader range of sound during group activities and class discussions.

For detailed information regarding the use of amplification in the educational setting, see Bess et al. (1981).

The Children Themselves

The children on whom this book is based have hearing losses that range from mild to profound. Few have had the benefit of early intervention in the area of language development. A number of the children have had limited exposure to English outside of school. Few have been taken to a public library or have ever been read to at home in any language.

Several children display classic signs of learning disabilities. In some instances, this appears to be a by-product of years of sensory and experiential deprivation.

The degree of hearing loss does not always bear a direct relationship to a child's success in school. Children who lose their hearing after beginning to develop language may be expected to have a foundation that is lacking in children who are prelingually deaf or hard of hearing. Children who wear amplification consistently at home as well as in school are receiving the feedback and reinforcement necessary for language acquisition. Middle ear infections cause additional hearing loss in some children, further limiting language development.

Even children with mild hearing losses, if language development has not been fostered, can display seemingly insurmountable lags in vocabulary, syntax, reading, and writing. In contrast, children whose learning needs have been consistently met, whether orally or through sign language, may come to participate fully in grade-level activities.

Chapter 4

Beginnings

Deaf and hard-of-hearing children enter the resource room with their individual patterns of strengths and weaknesses. One child has been wearing hearing aids for years, while another is just now being fitted with amplification. One child picks up language easily, while another has barely begun to understand and use everyday words.

In their earliest school days, children give hints as to who they are and the kinds of learners they will become. Looking back, it is fascinating and instructive to recognize traits, inclinations, and aptitudes that make themselves known from the very beginning.

The following vignettes illustrate ways in which three children revealed important aspects of themselves as learners during their first days and weeks of school.

CRYSTAL

Crystal, not quite six years old, brought to the resource room program a vocabulary of a few hundred words and a handful of two-word phrases.

Placing Crystal in kindergarten rather than first-grade gave her the setting she needed to expand her comprehension and use of language. In spite of a severe hearing loss, Crystal's hearing aid gave her a significant amount of usable hearing. Crystal, however, relied solely on visual and contextual cues.

23

Her hearing remained in the background, a jumble of sound that was easier to ignore. Help was needed before she could be expected to sort out the not quite comprehensible sounds being transmitted to her ear.

In order to focus Crystal's attention on her hearing, I began to cover my mouth with my hand while talking to her. This took away the crutch of speechreading and forced her to concentrate on what she was hearing. Crystal did not trust that she could make sense out of the sounds she heard. She strained to look under and behind my hand. I reassured her that she could understand me, and encouraged her to listen. I knew from her audiogram that what I was demanding of her was within reason.

Within two weeks, Crystal had begun to comprehend with ease. As I stopped covering my mouth, Crystal found her own blend of listening supported by visual cues, but without going back to her earlier tense and exclusive reliance on speechreading.

Crystal's new-found ability to use her hearing, imperfect though it was, boosted her language intake dramatically. Her vocabulary blossomed. Words led to phrases; phrases became sentences. Crystal's language acquisition was not confined to words gained through formal instruction.

From early on, Crystal's mother had spoken to her as one adult to another. This level of communication would have gone over the heads of most young deaf or hard-of-hearing children; but Crystal, a natural mimic, picked up chunks of language from these and other conversations. Her ability to retain and use language was exceptional. Crystal's speech contained errors typical of a child with her hearing loss: faulty articulation, missing grammatical and syntactical endings, and errors in verb tense. However, from the rate and effortlessness with which Crystal picked up language and made it her own, it was evident that she had a remarkable ear and flair for language.

A few months into kindergarten, Crystal revealed a capacity for abstract thinking and an ability to wrestle her thoughts into words in spite of her still-limited vocabulary. One afternoon at bus time, Crystal excitedly showed me her loose tooth and explained with a mixture of words and pantomime that "wings" was going to leave money under her pillow. "Oh, the tooth fairy's going to come!" I responded, giving her the words she was lacking. I had Crystal repeat what she had said, this time using the new words.

The next afternoon, Crystal wiggled her still-loose tooth and gave me another demonstration of how "wings" would come in through her bedroom window. "Wings!" I objected. I refreshed her memory and we retold the story together. I teased Crystal that I was going to tickle her the next time she said "wings."

The following morning, Crystal ran over to me in the lunchroom. There was a gap where her tooth had been, and her eyes were shining. Her mouth started to form the sound of "w. . . ." She stopped herself. The words eluded her. "You know . . ." she groped, furrowing her brow. "You know . . ." And then she burst out: "You know, like Jesus Christ!"

I was amazed that this little girl, with her bare-bones vocabulary and minimum of concepts and life experiences, had found this analogy to convey her thoughts. The tooth fairy and Jesus Christ: both more than human; both, for her, somewhere up in the sky. This language facility and drive to communicate her thoughts and feelings, which had their beginnings in these early days, were to characterize Crystal all the way through elementary school.

SHELLEY

As with all learners, temperament plays a part in the learning styles of deaf and hard-of-hearing children. Shelley, also starting kindergarten, was receiving her third year of speech and language support from a speech and hearing center. One day during the first week of school, I needed to call her family for a piece of information. Shelley was excited at the prospect of saying hello to her mother. The phone was at the back of a large desk, and Shelley had seated herself in the big office chair. Unable to reach the phone, she had begun to squirm discontentedly.

I let Shelley know that I realized she wanted to reach the phone. Using words and gestures, I asked her what she could do to make herself taller. She could have knelt or stood up; a thick Manhattan telephone book was on the desk within reach. None of these solutions suggested themselves to Shelley. I offered her broad hints. Her eyes glazed over and became vacant; the part of Shelley available for communication and learning had withdrawn before my eyes. Further encouragement met with crocodile tears. Shelley remained beyond reach for the rest of our session. A quick check with her speech therapist confirmed that this was a usual behavior pattern.

What Shelley did not show that day was the pleasant and even personality that was to be her hallmark throughout her elementary school years. This cheerful steadiness typically accompanied learning tasks that came easily to her. These were likely to be of a rote, repetitive nature. As time went on, Shelley's range of skills and abilities increased; but at any given stage, she resisted stretching her mind beyond her comfort level. Demands on her thinking continued to call forth the same withdrawal demonstrated that first week of school.

Enthusiasm tempered by the threat of withdrawal were present side by side as Shelley and I began our work together.

TOM

Not every child arrives in the resource room program at the beginning of his or her school life. Tom's hearing loss was not diagnosed until age seven. No English was spoken at home. Without hearing aids, Tom could hear only at very close range. He had managed to pick up his native language, and was said to speak with age-appropriate vocabulary, sentence structure, and fluency.

Tom had acquired virtually no English during his first three years of school in bilingual classes. He had begun to wear hearing aids during the last half of second grade. The optimum distance between speaker and hearing aid user is three feet. This almost certainly put the teacher beyond Tom's range of hearing for most of the day. In addition, "school talk" does not always meet the needs of a beginning language learner. Naming the varieties of apples purchased on a trip to the farmers' market, sharing stories and poetry, or discussing an imaginary trip through the solar system are stimulating and enriching activities for children with a language foundation, or for those who have no obstacles in the way of their acquiring a second language. Tom's hearing loss prevented him from picking up English in this incidental way.

Tom's family had visited the resource room at the end of second grade. In order to get a sense of the extent of his language delay, I took out a game of picture lotto. Picking up the first card, I described a picture of "a boy eating an apple." Tom was at a loss. I simplified the language. Tom did not recognize "apple," or any of the common words that followed. At age eight, spending a year in kindergarten was out of the question. I was alarmed at the thought of Tom's sitting through third grade with no English and an apparent difficulty in acquiring even basic vocabulary. I felt sure that Tom must have a language impairment in addition to his hearing loss. He had, after all, spent three years in partially English-speaking classrooms. I was convinced that regular third grade was an unfeasible placement.

I was right. Auditory and visual perception problems became evident as time went on. Each constituted a stumbling block to Tom's learning to speak, read, and write.

I was also wrong. I had not taken into account this boy's active intelligence and commitment to learning. Even with no one to reinforce his learning of English at home, Tom immediately began increasing his vocabulary by ten or twelve words a day. Tom was a science and history buff from early on. He molded his handful of words into questions of pressing concern: "Ms. Stelling! How birds fly?" "Ms. Stelling! Why thunder?"

As evidence of Tom's interests and abilities accumulated, I began to question my own uncertainty as to the reasonableness of this placement. I wondered whether the resource room could possibly give Tom the foundation he needed to succeed in the mainstream. It felt worth a try.

Chapter 5

The Reading-Language Link

WHY READING?

It is no coincidence that my reservations about Tom's ability to profit from the resource room program were dispelled as we inched our way through a humorous pre-primer story, with Tom slapping his thigh and chortling, "That [*sic*] funny, man!"

Researchers Michael Breene and Christopher Candlin (1980) believe that "just as no single communicative ability can really develop independently of the other abilities, so the development of any single skill may well depend on the appropriate development of the other skills. A refinement of the skill of reading, for example, will contribute to the refinement of the skill of speaking and vice-versa" (p. 95).

Tom savored words and phrases from these early stories, and integrated them into his own language with glee. His humor, as well as his earnest probing, revealed both his alert intelligence and the breadth of his interest. The language Tom needed to learn and communicate was coming to him primarily from reading, and from the dialogue that grew out of reading together.

Reading: A Resource Room Priority

E. A. Limbrick and others (1992) hypothesize that the relationship between language and reading is bi-directional. Their longitudinal study of 45 deaf children, some signing and some oral, finds a .90 correlation between language proficiency and reading performance.

The study points to growing up in a literate environment, one in which children are read to frequently, as a predictor of progress in reading. Harvard psychologist Jerome Kagan (1968) reports that reading to children and listening attentively to their responses play an important role in reversing verbal shortcomings in children who are lacking in language experience. Early literacy experiences are negligible for many deaf and hard-of-hearing children. This suggests that reading to children in the resource room is a crucial element in both their reading and their language development.

The authors (Limbrick et al. 1992) go on to state that the most powerful predictor of reading progress for school-age children, hearing and deaf alike, is the amount of time actually engaged in reading instruction. Growth in reading is closely tied to growth in language. For children who are deaf and hard of hearing, print compensates to some extent for auditory language-input deficits. Time devoted to reading is therefore inseparable from time allotted to language development. The reading-language link justifies giving reading a prominent place in the resource room period.

WHY LITERATURE?

Bettelheim (1989) discusses the need for the child's emotions, imagination, and intellect to support and enrich one another. This engenders the inner resources that endow children's lives with meaning, enabling them to believe that they will one day make an important difference in the world. In Bettelheim's eyes, two factors are most responsible for accomplishing this task. The first is the impact of parents and other care-givers. The second is children's literature.

Bettelheim maintains that, of all the arts, literature is closest to the human heart. It leads children toward awareness of others and of themselves. Bettelheim describes good literature as being precise, intelligent, and colorful. It offers children a model of the meaning, sensitivity, and language they need to express their thoughts and feelings clearly.

Bettelheim's view has a further implication. Good writing opens the way to good teaching. A bored teacher cannot teach with vitality. Works of literature survive repeated readings and rereadings. The beauty and meaning inherent in them are always fresh. Literature engages our own minds and hearts, enabling us to awaken the minds and hearts of our children.

BACK TO LANGUAGE

The following discussion of early language development is derived from Bruner (1983).

Research indicates that parents play "a far more active role in language acquisition than simply modeling the language and providing input" (p. 38). Peekaboo and other games of infancy provide familiar and repetitive contexts that aid parents and babies in forming and interpreting messages. Parents instinctively shape communicative interactions to their child's level, gradually raising their level of expectation while remaining attuned to the child's capacities. A mother discusses a story with her 23-month-old child:

Mother:	What's that?
Child:	Ouse.
Mother:	Mouse, yes. That's a mouse.
Child:	More mouse (pointing to another picture).
Mother:	No, those are squirrels. They're like mice but with long tails. Sort of.
Child:	Mouse, mouse, mouse.
Mother:	Yes, all right, they're mice.
Child:	Mice, mice (p. 86).

Mothers "often do not know what their children have in mind when they vocalize or gesture, nor are they sure their own speech has been understood by their children. But they are prepared to negotiate in the tacit belief that *something* comprehensible can be established" (p. 86). Children learn that using language involves attention and taking turns; they learn what is worth talking about and are helped to extend the words they know into new contexts. Bruner extends the theory that children are endowed with an innate capacity for language learning. He emphasizes that, in addition, linguistic competence depends on learning to use language by using it communicatively.

In the following exchange, Lizzie's mother collaborates in conversation with her two-and-one-half-year-old daughter:

Child:	I'm a Mummy.
Adult:	Lizzie's not a Mummy, is she?

Child (holding doll):   Gotta baby, I'm a Mummy.
Adult: Lizzie's got a pretend baby, so she's a pretend
          Mummy.
Child: I'm a Mummy, yes (p. 57).

Lizzie's mother employed a range of strategies aimed at developing her child's participation in their shared dialogue. She:

- queried what the child said;

- prompted Lizzie to enlarge on what she had said earlier and to clarify what she meant;

- offered positive feedback;

- expanded the child's utterances and provided a better sentence model; and

- introduced some missing information ("pretend Mummy") to develop what the child was intending to say (pp. 57–58).

In her role as language facilitator, Lizzie's mother was finely attuned to her child's needs as a "language novice" (p. 57). She gauged her daughter's level of understanding accurately. She interpreted what the child intended to say and made it explicit.

Boothroyd (1988) calls dialogue "the proper forum of language development" (p. 130). For deaf and hard-of-hearing children at an early stage of language development, the conversation incidental to a planned resource room activity may be as valuable a source of language learning as the activity itself:

Nancy: Puzzle . . .
Teacher: I want the puzzle.
Nancy: I want . . .
Teacher: I want . . . the puzzle.
Nancy: I want puzzle.
Teacher: Here you are. Here's the puzzle.
Nancy (holding her hands over her ears in anticipation):   Ow!
Teacher: It's going to be loud! Turn it over.
Nancy: Over . . .

READING, LANGUAGE, AND LIFE

Because children with hearing impairments do not acquire language as effortlessly as hearing children, it takes particular awareness to use language that is a step beyond what they already know. Overloading a conversation with unfamiliar words and grammatical or syntactical structures defeats this aim. Similarly, matching one's language too closely to the child's own level ensures comprehension without stimulating further language development. Learning to choose one's words in a way that balances these two needs is an essential skill for both parents and teachers if they are to be effective language educators.

Partly for this reason, many young resource room children have been exposed to a very narrow range of language outside of school. Limited language restricts children's experience of the world. Limbrick (1992) discusses a cumulative environmental lag caused by the fact that, unless directly engaged in communication, deaf and hard-of-hearing children are limited in their exposure to surrounding interactions.

For children in the early stages of language development, language evolves from shared experience. "Real-life" experiences cannot be easily or systematically duplicated in the resource room setting. Dialogue based on reading serves as a school equivalent of early parent-child interactions. The language of a well-chosen book is within the child's reach. At the same time, new words and concepts inevitably present themselves, both in the story itself and in ensuing discussions. Reading becomes a source of concepts that bring children increasingly in touch with the world around them.

Sculptor-author Anne Truitt (1984) reflects on mealtime as an important ceremony of family living:

> Where else can children learn so easily and pleasantly, and at such range when guests are included, what it is to be grown-up? The world of children is fascinating but very personal. The presence of adults in the full cry of conversation, with opinions, interests, engagements, and responsibilities discussed, crisscrossed by agreements and disagreements, laced with rhetoric, is so pungent with variety that children can learn without harm to their self-respect that they are, for all their interest to themselves, on their way to larger definitions (p. 63).

A story offers a concrete point of reference for a child who would be lost in a free-flowing conversation. As we read together in the resource room, we do more than increase reading competence. Equally important, we offer children glimpses of our world and theirs, and open their way to "larger definitions" of themselves.

Chapter 6

Structured and/or "Natural": A Closer Look

Because of the marked language deficits of children who are deaf and hard of hearing, natural or experiential language learning has long been the approach of choice for these children. Whole language, with its integrated approach to the teaching of reading and writing, embodies the essence of natural language learning.

Content and meaning are at the heart of the whole language or language experience philosophy; the nature and degree of structure built into individual activities vary from classroom to classroom. In working with children with language delays, nothing is more important than giving shape to every reading, writing, and language activity as it arises.

THE NEED FOR "SCAFFOLDING"

Adults who are familiar with young children's daily activities, likes and dislikes, and early attempts at language are able to comprehend what children are trying to say even before they are able to express themselves clearly. By understanding the world from the child's point of view, adults compensate for children's language limitations and ensure effective communication. Snow and Ninio (1986) note that no such "scaffolding" is available to children when they begin to read.

For children with language deficits, it is essential that parents and teachers continue to provide the scaffolding, or structure, that will enable children to comprehend and integrate new material in every area of learning. This entails knowing when to present an unfamiliar concept, pacing instruction to suit the child's needs, and keeping the background context as simple as possible in order to highlight new information. The more each communication "holds the attentional stage solo and does not share the child's limited attentional capacities with other attractions" (Kagan 1968, 82) the more effective the instructional intervention will be.

Activities designed to help children advance in language, reading, writing, and general knowledge are described throughout *The Words They Need*. The shaping of each activity reflects the interplay between the learning task and the child's instructional needs. The resulting structure becomes the vehicle by which concepts are quickly and deeply understood and integrated into "the child's own learning schema" (Kagan 1968, 82).

One aspect of structure, in the context of early reading instruction, is the systematic study of letter-sound associations, or phonics. Whether and how to incorporate phonics into the teaching of reading is open to interpretation within the whole language community.

READING INSTRUCTION: A HISTORICAL OVERVIEW

The value and prominence accorded to phonics as an element of reading instruction has fluctuated over the years. The following description of reading instruction in this century is condensed from Beck and Juel (1995, 24–25).

In the early 1900s, reading instruction typically consisted of extended syllable drill disconnected from meaningful context. By the 1930s, this method had been supplanted by the look-say or whole word method. The look-say approach fostered word recognition without analysis of word parts. Teachers found whole word learning easier and less tedious than emphasis on rote drill.

The look-say method remained the basis of reading instruction until challenged by Flesch in *Why Johnny Can't Read* (1955). Flesch's exhortation for a return to phonics was given credence by Chall (1967), who analyzed and interpreted research pointing to the benefits of early and systematic phonics instruction. The more recent evolution of whole language instruction, with its emphasis on engaging children's interests through meaningful and relevant learning experiences, has influenced every area of language learning.

READING DEFINED

Adams and Bruck (1993) describe the reading process:

> Skillful readers are found to march their eyes through all of the words of a sentence and then to pause at each period (Just and Carpenter 1987). It is during these end-of-sentence pauses that listeners or readers actively construct and reflect on their interpretations; it is during these interludes that they work out the collective meaning of the chain of words in memory and its contribution to their over-all understanding of the conversation or text. Yet, in order for this interpretive process to succeed, the whole clause or sentence must still exist, more or less intact, in the listener's or reader's memory when she or he is ready to work on it. The quality of this representation is highly dependent upon the speed and effortlessness of the word recognition process. If it takes too long or too much effort for the reader to get from one end of the sentence to the other, the beginning will be lost from memory before the end has been registered (p. 119).

This framework supports findings by numerous researchers that "poor word identification skills are strongly coupled with poor reading comprehension" (p. 119). Vellutino (1991) observes that "less than optimum facility in word identification drains off cognitive resources that would normally be devoted to comprehension processes, thereby impeding these processes" (p. 438). This position contrasts with that of whole language educators such as Smith (1985) and Goodman (1967). Goodman describes skillful readers as relying heavily on contextual clues while making minimal use of phonics information. According to Stanovich (1986), the truth of the notion that fluent readers rely more on context "is critically dependent on the distinction between the use of context as an aid to *word recognition* and its use to aid *comprehension processes*" (p. 366).

WHOLE LANGUAGE, PHONICS, AND THE HEARING-IMPAIRED CHILD

In analyzing the requirements of early reading instruction, Adams and Bruck (1993) point to a ready knowledge of letter sequences and spelling patterns as essential to processing words of "known meaning but incomplete visual familiarity"

(p. 119). Children who enter school with little phonemic aware-ness are likely to encounter particular difficulty reading and writing words not in their sight vocabularies.

The speech discrimination that enables children to make letter-sound associations is problematic for many children with impaired hearing. Dramatic improvement in listening ability can be achieved through amplification and auditory training. However, for most school-age children who have had little training of this kind before entering school, this is a long-range goal.

In addition, words of incomplete visual familiarity are likely to be of unknown meaning as well. When asked to reflect on her own reading strategies, a hearing first grader in a whole language classroom replied that it was hard to figure out a word if "you don't know that word" (Avery 1993, 340). While most kindergarteners are able to demonstrate comprehension of sophisticated language structures by making inferences and rephrasing long, syntactically complicated sentences (Beck and Juel 1995), hearing-impaired children of five, six, and even older may be at a loss to understand the most fundamental vocabu-lary in which the story is being unfolded. Their need for a meaning-centered approach to the development of language, reading, and writing has made whole or natural language learn-ing the traditional path to reading and writing.

In most whole language classrooms, whole word learning takes precedence over explicit phonics instruction. Reading based on sight vocabulary alone, while serviceable for begin-ning readers, may lead to difficulty at more advanced levels (Adams and Bruck 1995). Literate and articulate deaf adults at-test to the possibility of achieving competence in reading with little, if any, knowledge of phonics. Yet the fourth-grade reading level of the average deaf seventeen-year old (Center for Assess-ment and Demographic Studies 1991) indicates that highly liter-ate deaf adults are the exception rather than the rule.

Phonics and Whole Language: A Synthesis

Adams (1991) believes that whole language and phonics are not mutually exclusive, but are concerned with two differ-ent issues within the domain of beginning reading. She reasons that to treat whole language "as an issue of phonics versus no phonics is not only to misrepresent it, but to place all of its valuable components at genuine risk" (p. 51).

Adams views whole language as . . .

> an acknowledgement that there is more to reading than phonics; and through such activities as read-alouds, big-book sharing, language experience, and creative writing, it is an effort to invite active exploration and appreciation of its many dimensions. It is a reaction to mindless worksheets . . . to boring, overly controlled stories . . . to compartmentalization of instruction. . . . Both theory and research indicate with unqualified force that . . . [integration across the curriculum] is incredibly important for productive education (p. 51).

At the same time, the author regards whole language learning as "strictly independent from issues of the nature of the knowledge and processes involved in reading and learning to read" (p. 52).

Once word recognition catches up to their language skill, most beginning readers are able to read stories that match the sophistication of their expressive vocabularies, concepts, and knowledge. In contrast, the language of young readers who are deaf and hard of hearing may be almost as limited as their ability to recognize words in print. Hearing-impaired children require knowledge that will give them access to the printed word, while building an underlying language foundation that will render words meaningful.

As part of this process, there appears to be every reason to give those children with sufficient hearing the means of learning letter-sound correspondences. Instruction that increases fluency and accuracy and gives children access to words that are not yet in their sight vocabulary cannot help but enhance comprehension as well. Here, phonics and whole language meet, each contributing to children's development as readers and writers.

Chapter 7

Toward Reading

Wilbur was merely suffering the doubts and fears that often go with finding a new friend. In good time he was to discover that he was mistaken about Charlotte. Underneath her rather bold and cruel exterior, she had a kind heart, and she was to prove loyal and true to the very end.

E. B. White, *Charlotte's Web*

"Broken."

Douglas, age 6

Most young children bring a rich and versatile language foundation to their earliest school experiences. The reading aloud of *Charlotte's Web* (White 1952) has become a yearly tradition in at least one first-grade classroom (Avery 1993). With their hearts and imaginations stirred, Avery's young listeners are well on their way to reading. Learning to decode will take them deeper and deeper into a world of language and literature which is, in part, already theirs.

The extent of a child's vocabulary, syntax, story knowledge, and appreciation of the sounds of language determine the choice of early reading material. Children who are deaf or hard of hearing are likely to have significant deficits in each of these areas. This chapter addresses the process of selecting beginning reading material that accommodates children's language delays, while providing scope for further language development.

41

FIRST STEPS IN LANGUAGE

Reading is only as meaningful as the understanding a child brings to the printed word. Experiences that engender context-related language constitute all children's earliest reading lessons. This kind of language input comes naturally to parents of normally hearing children. A baby's responsiveness to voices, a toddler's understanding and imitation of words and connected language—these provide the encouragement parents need to continue the talking and expectation of talking that stimulate language development.

In the beginning, parents of young deaf and hard-of-hearing children lack this feedback to guide them. Yet preschoolers with limited hearing are no different from hearing children in their need for experiential and verbal stimulation. As with all children, parents need to gear their language input to the child's level and a bit beyond, bringing him or her to the point of imitating and eventually using language spontaneously. Every word gained in this way increases the language foundation available when the child begins to read.

Speech and language therapists in hospital clinics and other specialized settings are experienced in working with hearing-impaired infants and preschoolers. It is the task of these professionals to give parents the support and knowledge required to begin the process of language development. Because *The Words They Need* addresses the learning needs of school-age children, the earliest stages of language intervention are beyond the scope of this book. For a detailed description of the language needs of deaf and hard-of-hearing preschool children and how to meet them, see Boothroyd (1988).

STORY ELEMENTS AND THE BEGINNING READER

Snow and Ninio (1986, 119–20) identify the ability to understand and produce language that is a step removed from the immediate experience as the most difficult and most critical prerequisite to literacy. This ability has its roots in the child's earliest reading experiences. As parents and toddlers read the same picture book over and over, the core vocabulary is repeated and extended. In time, the focus shifts from labeling the people and objects depicted on the page, to discussing precursors and consequences of the event.

As children's acquaintance with stories broadens, they learn to use their prior experiences or knowledge to construct "expectations" about what is likely to occur in a story (Stein and Trabasso 1982, 215). The more closely a story fits an expected structure, the easier it is for the child—first as listener, then as reader—to grasp and remember the important ideas:

Setting: 1. Once there was a big grey fish named Albert.
2. He lived in a big icy pond near the edge of a forest.
Initiating Event: 3. One day, Albert was swimming around the pond.
4. Then he spotted a big juicy worm on the top of the water.
Internal Response: 5. Albert knew how delicious worms tasted.
6. He wanted to eat that one for his dinner.
Attempt: 7. So he swam very close to the worm.
8. Then he bit into him.
Consequence: 9. Suddenly Albert was pulled through the water into a boat.
10. He had been caught by a fisherman.
Reaction: 11. Albert felt sad.
12. He wished he had been more careful (p. 219).

Story "structure" refers to the way ideas in the story are connected. In a well-formed children's story, characters are placed in settings; they have goals that are expressly stated or can be inferred. Characters make plans or undertake actions to achieve these goals. Actions unfold in an orderly sequence, and lead to outcomes that provoke emotional reactions in children (Anderson et al. 1985).

A sound structure makes it easier for readers to connect parts of the story. Understanding "which . . . aspects of the situation are relevant, and the kinds of interrelations among them that deserve attention" (Adams and Bruck 1993, 122) is basic to the knowledge required for meaningful reading.

Two additional factors influence the choice of beginning reading material. First, children are more likely to comprehend a text that conforms to their own speech patterns, as opposed to sentences written in styles they seldom hear or use. Second, children receiving systematic phonics instruction need experience reading words that reinforce spelling patterns as they are introduced.

The Young Deaf or Hard-of-Hearing Reader

Many deaf and hard-of-hearing children enter school lacking in vocabulary, phonemic awareness, and exposure to stories. Giving these children "*all* of the elements necessary for constructing meaning" (Anderson et al. 1985, 44) may mean going back to the labeling stage until children acquire a core vocabulary and begin to express themselves in words, phrases, and simple sentences.

The importance of children's knowledge of story structure as a basis for success in reading leads Anderson to suggest using stories that are partly understood, or even partly known by heart, as a natural strategy for getting a child started in reading. For children who lack the language and knowledge on which to base story selection, the language-experience story becomes an invaluable means of language development, as well as an introduction to reading itself.

Like parents' sensitively timed input into their babies' early language learning, the language-experience story is carefully fitted to the child's own level of language and knowledge. At a stage at which language development and reading are inseparable, I have found that nothing compares with stories that grow out of the child's own experience, narrated in the child's own words, as a vehicle for fostering reading-language development.

THE LANGUAGE-EXPERIENCE APPROACH TO READING

"Look, Ms. Stelling," announced Douglas as we stepped outside his kindergarten classroom on the way to the resource room. Douglas was a severely hard-of-hearing six-year-old whose mother had been optimistic that her son's language delays and inconsistent responses to sounds were within normal limits. For that reason, Douglas' hearing loss had been only recently diagnosed. Now that he was wearing hearing aids, he was beginning to pick up words and phrases for the first time. Douglas lifted his arm to show me his new toy watch. Its hands jiggled loosely as he flapped his wrist. "Broken," he lamented.

In the resource room, I took out chart paper and a marker. "Remember you showed me your watch?" I asked, holding up my arm just as Douglas had done. "Remember you said, 'Look, Ms. Stelling'?" I imitated his rueful expression and intonation. I picked up the marker and wrote each word, reading as I wrote. I went back to the beginning, underlining the words with my finger. I invited Douglas to read with me. We read together once or twice. I wondered aloud whether Douglas could put his finger under the first word and follow along as we read. He was able to do this.

Next I asked Douglas to let me see his watch. He took it off and handed it to me. Glancing back and forth between the watch and the paper, I carefully drew a circle and two horizontal bands. "What happened?" I asked sympathetically. "Broken," he explained once again. I added two dangling hands, then recorded the word "broken" under the drawing. We read together as we had done before.

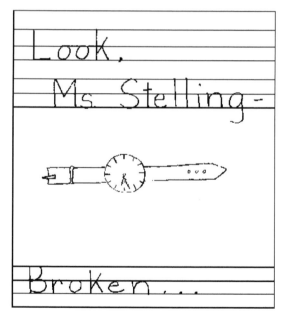

After taping the story to the wall, I gave Douglas a fresh sheet of paper. He copied the words and picture as best he could, and we read his version together before folding it up for him to take home. Thus ended Douglas' first formal reading lesson.

Parents and teachers facilitate children's use of language by providing ongoing opportunities for producing language. As frequently as needed, we assist children in communicating what they have to say.

Experience stories provide opportunities for the development of attention, memory, vocabulary, reading readiness, reading comprehension, and the understanding and use of connected language. Along with other activities, experience stories form a scaffold that enables children to participate actively in the acquisition of language essential to reading.

DEVELOPING SIGHT VOCABULARY

The process of learning to decode is not much different for children who are deaf and hard of hearing than it is for beginning readers in general. All children need to develop sight vocabulary. All children benefit from learning basic word attack skills. Hearing loss is not an obstacle to word recognition. Deaf and hard-of-hearing children have no particular difficulty acquiring and retaining sight vocabulary.

Douglas proudly took his story home with him that afternoon. The next day, we recalled what had happened, and reread the original version together. As Douglas watched, I wrote out a sentence strip to match each sentence in his story. For this activity I used lined oaktag—sturdy paper available in rolls or as precut "sentence strips."

During the next few days, Douglas showed that reading stories came easily to him. Matching sentence to sentence was not a problem. One day, I took a sentence strip he had just read, and cut it apart:

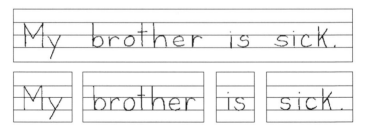

Douglas recognized the words, and had no trouble rearranging them to form the original sentence. He was able to do this with numerous sentences over the next several days.

At this point, I transferred every word from Douglas' three or four stories to construction paper flashcards. From then on, new words were printed on flashcards as they came up, and reviewed daily. This gave Douglas a small but solid sight vocabulary. (Vocabulary expansion through reading is discussed in detail in Chapter 11.)

DEVELOPING PHONEMIC AWARENESS

Word attack skills play a part in facilitating word recognition. Deaf and hard-of-hearing children are capable of associating sounds with letters and blending them into words to the extent that their hearing and auditory discrimination allow. Recognizing sound-symbol associations goes hand in hand with the development of sight vocabulary.

With the youngest children, I sometimes tack envelopes representing various sounds on the bulletin board. In the beginning, I select sounds that contrast clearly with one another. The phonemes /b/, /l/, and /sh/ are highly visible on the lips, and easily distinguishable in their manner of production. They are acoustically different and easy to hear, even for children with significant hearing loss.

On small cards, I draw pictures of familiar objects beginning with each sound:

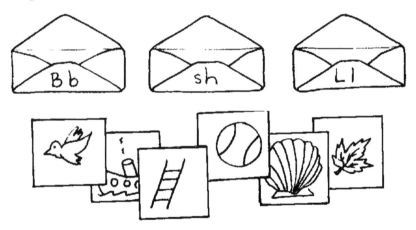

With the help of these cards, children learn to answer two questions: "What sound does *mitten* begin with?" and "What letter makes the sound of /m/?" Sorting pictures into envelopes is an activity that children enjoy. It consolidates basic vocabulary, develops auditory discrimination, clarifies articulation, and introduces initial consonants. Children's recognition of initial consonants carries over into reading.

Once children begin amassing sight vocabulary, it does not take long before they have several words beginning with the same consonant:

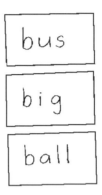

This provides the opportunity to draw children's attention to final consonants, and to begin differentiating among words on that basis.

At this early stage, phonics is closely allied with language acquisition. Children's own language constitutes the primary source of words used to introduce sounds and blending. Once children have mastered a dozen or so sounds and have begun to blend those sounds, they are able to benefit from the same kinds of activities that help any child acquire word attack skills. (Exploring phonics instruction with children who are deaf and hard of hearing is described more fully in Chapter 19.)

BRINGING MEANING TO READING

Language-experience stories provide a starting point for developing sight vocabulary and phonemic awareness. However, for children who cannot yet comprehend or express themselves in connected language, these skills are of limited value.

For this reason, the skills-related value of experience stories pales in comparison with their role in developing the language that will bring children closer to reading with comprehension. Stories such as the tale of Douglas' watch parallel the process of normal language acquisition. They impart value to moments of importance in a child's life, and honor the language in which they are conveyed. The process of drawing a salient feature of each story with just enough recognizable detail rivets children's attention, and contributes to their identification with the story. Eliciting experiences and recording them in words and pictures gives children an emotional investment in their stories, and in the process of reading and writing. The language and memory cues provided by the children's own language contribute to success in reading. Above all, experience stories affirm children as users of language as they reflect upon their own words and thoughts.

As stories accumulate, children gain facility in communicating the day-to-day happenings of their lives. At this point, the language-experience story becomes a vehicle for taking their language a step further. Parents naturally extend their toddler's single-word utterances by modeling back more complete phrases and sentences. Experience stories can be used to provide similar feedback. As time went on, Douglas' "broken" grew to "My watch—broken" and, eventually, to "My watch is broken." Intangible bits of language ranging from "is" and "the" to more sophisticated grammatical and syntactical concepts can be incorporated into experience stories as children show signs of readiness.

FROM EXPERIENCE STORIES TO BOOKS: A TRANSITION

Boothroyd (1988) discusses the interdependence of cognition and language. He speaks of adequate cognitive development as a prerequisite for language development; language, in turn, promotes further cognitive development. Without language, a child's cognitive development must remain at a primitive, concrete level. It is language that "frees people from the limitations of the immediate and the familiar. Language provides access to a world which can extend backwards and forwards in time and outward in space. Language gives the individual access to the accumulated experience of human society" (p. 29).

Experience stories help children acquire a language base. They could long remain a rich source of material for language and reading development. Yet as children gain a reading-language foundation, it becomes important to expand the scope of their reading.

Books stimulate children's minds and imaginations by leading them beyond the narrower, more self-focused realm of stories based on personal experience. "Real" stories bring socially aware deaf and hard-of-hearing youngsters into the circle of the regular classroom and age-appropriate reading. Whereas most children bring a knowledge of story structure to their first encounters with print, reading itself may serve to introduce the deaf or hard-of-hearing child to story shape and structure.

STUMBLING BLOCKS TO READING

"Bear waited for a while, then he poked his head up. When he did, the moon was right there looking at him."
Moongame (Asch 1984)

"I can find Clifford, no matter where he hides. We play camping out, and I don't need a tent. He can do tricks, too."
Clifford the Big Red Dog (Bridwell 1963)

"I have walked home from school alone before. I do it almost every day. But today it is different. Today my mother started working all day."
Home Alone (Schick 1980)

"In the great green room
There was a telephone
And a red balloon
And a picture of–
The cow jumping over the moon."
Goodnight Moon (Brown 1947)

The level of vocabulary, grammar, and syntax contained even in stories written for very young children places them beyond the reach of many deaf and hard-of-hearing beginning readers. In *Moongame*, a bear cub plays hide-and-seek with the moon, which has disappeared behind a cloud. The simplicity and directness of the illustrations and story line delight young children. Children who are deaf and hard of hearing can also appreciate the events and feelings of the story if told through the pictures rather than from the text. Two randomly chosen sentences include several words and phrases that are likely to be unfamiliar (*poked, right there, for a while*). Past tense, subordinate clauses, and gerunds make comprehension difficult.

Like most picture books, *Clifford the Big Red Dog* contains vocabulary and language structures that will probably be unfamiliar to children with limited language. While hearing children chuckle at Clifford's escapades, Emily's tongue-in-cheek commentary is likely to elude young deaf and hard-of-hearing children, who are left with illustrations that convey relatively scanty and disjointed information.

In *Home Alone*, a child describes his first afternoon at home by himself while his mother is at work. Past, present perfect, and future tenses are used throughout the book. Though the story is aimed at beginning readers, somewhat long and complex sentences are interspersed with simpler sentences. Even as a read-aloud, this story is too general and too abstract for children whose language level ties them to the here and now.

A beloved children's story contains difficulties for deaf and hard-of-hearing children at an early stage of language development. Much of the charm of *Goodnight Moon* comes from Margaret Wise Brown's subtle rhyme and lilting rhythm, her allusions to folk tales and nursery rhymes, and from the soft echo of words and phrases that linger in the ear. Many young children who are deaf and hard of hearing have yet to be exposed to "Hey, Diddle Diddle" or "The Three Bears"; their sensitivity to the nuances of language has yet to be developed. For them, experiencing *Goodnight Moon* becomes an exercise in pointing out and naming familiar objects in the illustrations.

FIRST THINGS FIRST

It took eight weeks for Kathy Robinson to develop the language that would render the opening sentence of *Peter Pan* meaningful to her two young deaf daughters (see Chapter 1). Two factors contributed to the success of this undertaking. First, Robinson made abstract concepts concrete by means of first-hand experiences that included several day trips and culminated in an overnight excursion. Second, these focused experiences constituted only one part of a daily life rich in language learning.

Families who are actively involved in the language development of their deaf and hard-of-hearing children have at their disposal opportunities not available in the resource room setting. Neither time nor distance presented an obstacle to Robinson's acquainting her children with a town, a village, and the city of London. At the same time, basic grammar, syntax, and vocabulary were continuously evolving from everyday activities. This combination gave the girls the language and experiences they needed to appreciate the adventures of Peter Pan with occasional clarification, once the difficulties presented by the opening sentence had been overcome.

What Robinson achieved as a teacher-mother at home needs to be accomplished differently in the more restricted resource room environment. Here, many children depend on the daily 45-minute session for most of their language learning. Devoting weeks of time and effort to the comprehension of a single sentence, or even a single story, comes at the expense of building a language foundation related to the child's immediate experience. The amount of clarification required to bring much of children's literature within the reach of a young deaf or hard-of-hearing child who lacks a substantial language foundation would eclipse the stories themselves, without necessarily rendering them accessible to the child. Many concepts cannot easily be made understandable at this point because they are too many steps removed from the child's own language level.

LOOKING FURTHER

Robinson's preschool age daughters needed to learn to listen with comprehension. Young resource room children, whose language may be at least equally delayed, are faced with the additional challenge of learning to read. For them, reading needs to be closely tied to language development.

The blending of reading and language characterizes whole language classrooms such as Avery's (1993). From September on, each of Avery's first graders selects reading books from the classroom library without regard to the level of the text. In individual mini-conferences lasting no more than a minute, Avery elicits and offers information and strategies to help children past stumbling blocks.

An independent and/or self-selected reading program such as Avery's cannot offer typical deaf and hard-of-hearing beginning readers the input they need as they stand on the verge of moving beyond experience stories. Even a more teacher-directed whole language setting using a more controlled progression of reading material cannot match the needs of six-year-old Douglas and other children who are still using single words to express complete thoughts. Such children cannot yet avail themselves of sound and language-based context clues. Something is needed that will meet them at their language level and take them a bit beyond, one step at a time.

Examining a Structured Reading Program

A structured reading series suggests itself as a possible answer to the language-reading needs of children with hearing impairments. Yet the following examination of one such series reveals that this program, while well tailored to the needs of children with age-appropriate language, is not tailored to the requirements of young deaf and hard-of-hearing children in several important ways. The same is likely to be true of other programs designed for typical beginning readers.

A product of New Zealand whole language education, the *Sunshine* series (Cowley 1986) is one example of a deliberately structured approach to introducing reading. Cutting [1990] outlines salient features of the program, which includes a wide range of beginning readers. The booklets provide a quantity of material that most children can read easily. Stories are written in the "natural language" children expect to hear. Each text introduces just enough challenge to encourage trying and to promote a willingness to solve problems. The readers form a developmental sequence. The reading banquet offered by this series is carefully considered and controlled. The stories are characterized by picture cues, repetition, and clarity of format. Sentence length expansion and the introduction of questions and dialogue are deliberately paced.

Repetitive language patterns play a key role in getting children started in reading with a minimum of adult intervention. The earliest booklets contain one or two sentences per page, accompanied by an illustration that clarifies the text:

- An orange
  An apple
  An umbrella . . . (*Huggles Can Juggle*)

- He eats,
  He drinks,
  He splashes . . . (*Little Brother*)

- In go some snails.
  In go some feathers.
  In go some thistles . . . (*Yuck Soup*)

- When she plays, she plays.
  When she sings, she sings.
  When she slides, she slides . . . (*Our Granny*)

- There are 7 clocks in Uncle Buncle's house.

There are 6 dogs in Uncle Buncle's house.
There are 5 TV's in Uncle Buncle's house . . . (*Uncle Buncle's House*)

- I like ice cream in the car.
I like ice cream in the plane.
I like ice cream in the snow . . . (*Ice Cream*)

- A hug is as warm as a hot water bottle.
A hug is as warm as a fur coat.
A hug is as warm as a stove . . . (*A Hug Is Warm*)

In summary, the *Sunshine* readers are based on the premise that children's own language ability enables them to make accurate word predictions. By reading aloud, teachers put the message of the booklets in children's heads. Children are then taught how to use picture, sound, and language cues to decipher the text. Cutting observes that the accessibility of the language of the readers enables children to read for themselves as early as the first day of school. This interplay between guided and independent reading is built into the program from the very beginning.

The Search Continues

To children with a developed ear and memory for language, and who are well grounded in the language of everyday life, the *Sunshine* series and similar booklets offer a carefully thought out pathway to reading. To say that many young deaf and hard-of-hearing children lack the prerequisites needed to pick up reading in this way is an understatement.

Sunshine readers contain some of the same stumbling blocks as do children's stories in general. In the examples cited above, it would probably be necessary to excerpt and clarify at least such words as *snails, feathers, thistles, slides, hot water bottle,* and *fur*. It is confusing to introduce words ending in "s" in the third person singular (Tim walks; Maria eats) to children who are unaware of this grammatical ending in other people's speaking, do not use it in their own, and may not yet be familiar with the root word. *There are* is likely to lack meaning to many children at this stage. Subordinate clauses, e.g., "When he eats, he eats . . ." are unfathomable to children who do not yet comprehend and use simple sentences. It is likely to take several years of language experience to bring children to the point of being able to grasp abstract concepts of the nature of "as . . . as."

Stumbling blocks notwithstanding, some young deaf and hard-of-hearing children are capable of the kind of rote reading that characterizes the early *Sunshine* booklets. These children gain from exposure to rhyme, cadence, and repetitive language patterns. For them, as for all children, it is important to build confidence in the use of contextual cues and willingness to take risks at guessing meanings. For hearing-impaired beginning readers who are ready, books of this nature offer these opportunities to the extent that the children's language allows. Even so, there is real reason to look further for a primary source of early reading material.

Whimsy: Pros and Cons

For six-year-old Nancy, learning to join in the chorus of "Clang, clang, rattle bing bang . . ." (see page 68) was an important step in the early stages of language acquisition. Because she had begun wearing hearing aids only months before entering school, this was Nancy's first experience with rhyme, rhythm, and the playful use of language. Her pleasure was obvious.

Whimsical language and settings engage the interest of beginning readers. These same characteristics, however, do not constitute the best starting point for children who are embarking on reading just as they are learning to formulate simple sentences related to concrete experiences. For children with limited language, reading and language development are inextricably intertwined. At this stage, deaf and hard-of-hearing children cannot afford to spend most of their time on texts that do not contribute to the development of connected language, however delightful or affecting a story may be to children at a more advanced stage of language development. Included are stories that are reduced to mere exercises in vocabulary because of a child's inability to appreciate rhyme, subtle humor, or other nuances of language. This holds equally true for the early *Sunshine* readers and for a children's classic such as *Goodnight Moon*.

Getting Closer

Stories that parallel children's real-life experiences and are conveyed in clear, everyday language have seemed to me particularly suited to meeting the need of young deaf and hard-of-hearing children for language development. Whimsical texts without a story line, while invaluable in other ways, do not lend themselves to discussions that draw on and extend children's abilities to understand and to express themselves. Similarly, descriptive language, even when vocabulary is simple and sentence structure clear, is less valuable than dialogue for children who need to learn to "tell" before they can tell "about."

A basal reading series comes close to meeting the language-learning needs of resource room beginning readers, whatever their ages. *Bears, Balloons,* and *Boats* (Durr et al. 1983) begin with two and three-word sentences in dialogue format. New words are introduced gradually but steadily; previously presented words are continuously reinforced.

The first story is six pages long. It begins with three sentences composed of four different words. By the last page, three additional words have been introduced. In the story, entitled "I Will Go," several birds discuss whether or not to enter a birdhouse. The maverick among them opts for the hollow of a tree, only to encounter a squirrel in residence. The script of this drama begins:

"I will go. Will you go?
I will go.

We will go. Will you go?
I will not go.

We will go.
You go. I will not go . . ."

Two stories later, a boy whose shoelace has come loose approaches a series of grown-ups, asking: "Can you help me? I can not get it to go in." Each time, something else causes the lace to come undone. A classmate's encouragement results in the little boy's proudly telling his mother: "Do not do it for me. I can do it. You will see."

The eighth and last story of the first primer shows a little fox about to enter a blueberry patch: "You can help me, Bear. I want to get a big surprise. The surprise is for Mother and Father."

Neither the language nor the plots of these little tales have the earmarks of great literature. But these stories, and those that follow, evoke laughter, concern, and enthusiasm for reading in young deaf and hard-of-hearing children. Their vocabulary, grammar, and syntax lend themselves to being incorporated into children's own language in a way that the language of literature ranging from *Charlotte's Web* to *Goodnight Moon* cannot.

BREAKING AWAY

I have regularly worked with children through the pre-primers and the first two or three readers in this series. At this point, I attempt to help children make the transition to regular picture books. But no method or philosophy can shorten the road to language acquisition faced by deaf and hard-of-hearing children. Three preprimers, two or three controlled readers, countless read-alouds, and a vast quantity of other language work can only begin the process of language development. Limited language continues to present overwhelming obstacles to reading.

The language facility manifested by Crystal in the tooth fairy incident (see pp. 24–25) continued to blossom, enabling her to read *Trumpet of the Swan* (White 1970) by the middle of third grade. This she accomplished independently and with excellent comprehension. Of all the children, only Crystal surged ahead on her own. Yet bit by bit, children read first one carefully selected book, then another. Each book brought them closer to being able to pick up a book of their choice without needing an adult guide to ensure their comprehension and facilitate their enjoyment of reading.

For children with few words and little connected language at their command, experience stories play an important part in language and reading development. No reading material is as easily adapted to the individual child's language level and experiential background.

As children gain a foundation in language and reading, other kinds of reading material broaden the scope of their learning in ways that experience stories cannot. Chall (1967) names folk tales and fairy tales as her personal preference for first and second graders. She states that she has never found a child who could not identify with such stories as *Cinderella, The Gingerbread Boy,* or *The Three Little Pigs.* Chall (1967) attributes this to the fact that these tales contain "struggle and triumph, right and wrong, laughter and tears—themes that have disappeared from modern stories based on familiar experiences" (pp. 311–12). Once grounded in the language of experience stories, children who are deaf and hard of hearing have the same need as all children for the language expansion and emotional richness inherent in folk tales, fairy tales, and other works of literature.

In primers that meet the needs of children with delayed language, many stories are themselves adaptations of folk and fairy tales. Others contribute to the language and knowledge of story structure that children need in order to comprehend stories a step removed from their personal experience.

For older beginning readers, maturation and inner language become factors in the selection of reading material. At first glance, experience stories appear more age appropriate and more relevant for a child such as Tom, who entered the resource room program at age eight with a severe hearing loss and no knowledge of English. Yet Tom, with barely enough words to understand even a preprimer story, gleefully inched his way through sentence after sentence, exploding with laughter as Frog leans out the window and empties a bucket of water on the heads of Fox and Bear for disturbing his slumber. A solid knowledge of his home language had given Tom an age-appropriate understanding of abstract concepts. This provided a foundation on which reading and language could develop.

" . . .That Tenuous Balance"

Fernald (1943) stresses using, from the beginning, reading material suited in terms of vocabulary and content to the child's intellectual level rather than to his or her reading skill. She maintains that the child is "much more interested in writing and reading fairly difficult material that is on the level of his understanding than simple material which is below his mental age level" (p. 44). Fernald drew this conclusion from her work with dyslexic children whose language, in spite of difficulties with reading and spelling, was unimpaired. Delayed language introduces another dimension to the teaching of reading and the choice of reading material. Age, level of language comprehension, and grasp of abstract concepts determine the most profitable approach to reading.

Based on her observations of children engaged in learning to read, Chall (1967) concludes that it was *"what the teacher did* with the method, the materials, and the children rather than the method itself that seemed to make the difference" (p. 270). Chall found children's interest to be "highly related to pacing—how instruction is geared to that tenuous balance between ease and difficulty for the child." Our informed selection of reading material for beginning deaf and hard-of-hearing readers is an important element in achieving this balance.

Moving Toward Literature

In an article about children who have experienced failure as readers, Carbo (1987) reports that thousands of profiles reveal most poor readers as "whole-to-part" learners (p. 198). These children respond to holistic teaching methods and high-interest materials that involve them emotionally.

My experience coincides with Carbo's findings. The road that has led to success in reading has been largely interest oriented, with skills playing a vital but supporting role in helping children gain access to the message of the book. Children's own leanings toward books of literary merit has become apparent as children gain independence in reading and begin to make their own selections.

Chapter 8

Forging Ahead in Reading

"I finally found it—a book I can't stop reading! The way this author writes, she doesn't let you put it down for a minute." With these words, eleven-year-old Crystal reveals her enthusiasm as a reader and the beginnings of a critical, evaluative sense. Both have emerged as Crystal's experience as a reader has broadened and deepened. This has been long in coming.

For years I had been attempting to combine the naturalness and spontaneity of the whole language approach with the structure needed to remediate language deficits. Yet the children's progress had remained discouragingly slow for too long.

Years of working on language and reading skills had brought a group of older children to the point of being able to read and enjoy simple books. The transition to more sophisticated picture books or to chapter books (children's novels) was not happening naturally. The twin obstacles of language and reading seemed overwhelming. Seeing fourth- and fifth-grade children still limited to the easiest of picture books with no sign of moving forward had become a source of frustration.

Children's novels differ from one another in several respects. Some are short, others long. In some, both vocabulary and dialogue closely parallel children's everyday language. In others, the proportion of description to dialogue increases, as vocabulary and syntax approach the level of adult language.

Around the time that I was becoming concerned with the children's lack of progress in reading, I discovered a number of short, clear chapter books with relatively simple texts. I resolved to help the children cross the bridge to age-appropriate reading by means of stories such as these.

THE CHILD'S FIRST BOOK

Anna Gillingham, remedial reading pioneer in the field of dyslexia, reflects on the choice of a child's first real reading book.

> The selection of the first book is of vital importance and is the teacher's responsibility, seldom to be relegated to the pupil. An expert guide employed to lead a tenderfoot through a wild region does not ask him to choose from a maze of unknown trails. The boy cannot evaluate his own skills and he does not know the books. On the other hand, after several weeks of close observation and companionship, the teacher, in her role of skilled guide, knows the boy's chief difficulties and major interests. Also, she can read the book and know in advance its probable pitfalls. At no time is her skill more on trial than in this fitting of book to boy.
>
> It is the teacher's first task to place in her pupil's hands a book fitted to his difficulties and interests. It is her continuing responsibility to prepare him to meet new difficulties and so to widen his interests . . . These students have been deprived of so much by their handicap that whatever they are helped to read should be a real contribution to their mental and emotional life, not a mere exercise for the sake of reading.
>
> The teacher must make the book a success. She may even do some of the reading herself, paraphrase some sentences as she goes. The selection must not be allowed to drag. The experience must be arresting as nothing has ever been before. Vivid description, plot development, portrayal of character—must all be discussed and enjoyed as in the hands of any other literature teacher (Gillingham and Stillman 1965, 128).

In selecting a child's first book after months of careful preparation, Gillingham is guided by two factors: the content must appeal to the child's interests; and the material must ensure success.

Many deaf and hard-of-hearing children about to embark on "real" reading are even less ready than dyslexic children at the same crossroad. Once Gillingham's student succeeds in decoding words and sentences, comprehension is likely to follow. For children who are deaf and hard of hearing, comprehension can be as major a deficit area as word knowledge.

No story is likely to be a perfect match for a given child's knowledge of phonics or sight vocabulary. Gillingham employs whatever adaptations are needed to bring the story to life and make the reading task attainable by the child. My hope was to do this for Curtis as he set out to read his first chapter book.

The book I selected was *The Chalkbox Kid* (Bulla 1987). It is the story of a young boy who turns down his share of flower seeds at school, knowing that he has no garden in which to plant them. In its place he finds a box of chalk and creates his own garden on the charred walls of a burned-out building. Curtis, the reader-to-be, was a sensitive and highly artistic fourth-grade boy with a moderate hearing loss.

Deficits in vocabulary, decoding, and language concepts made the going far more difficult than I had anticipated. I felt I was dragging Curtis through the usual combination of oral and silent reading, questioning, and discussion. Even short chapters proved tedious. The alternative to plodding along was going back to a more comfortable reading level. I was not willing to consider that option. My usual inclination is to be guided by a child's own readiness. This time, however, I was committed to moving Curtis and other children into the realm of chapter books and toward grade-level reading.

Educational researcher Lev Vygotsky interprets this dilemma in theoretical terms. He speaks of the child's "actual developmental level" as determined by the child's ability to carry out a task independently. Piaget (1968) believes that this level is dependent on maturation, and that teacher input must be geared to the child's readiness by giving children material they can handle without difficulty. Vygotsky, in contrast, sees beyond this stage to the "potential developmental level" at which problem solving becomes possible with adult guidance (Vygotsky 1962). The area between the child's actual developmental level and his or her potential level is termed by Vygotsky the "Zone of Proximal Development." It was this distance, applied to reading, that the children and I negotiated together.

"My Turn, Your Turn"

In order to rescue Curtis from discouragement, I began reading aloud with him, alternating sentences. This strategy had been suggested by a colleague as being valuable for children whose attention wanders. While this was not Curtis' problem, I decided to give it a try.

This "my turn, your turn" approach yielded immediate results. It moved our reading along at an interesting and satisfying pace. It took the drudgery out of decoding, since Curtis had to struggle with only one sentence at a time before sitting back and listening to mine.

It also furthered important fundamental needs in several areas. Our shared experience stimulated the dialogue that Boothroyd (1988) designates "the proper forum for language development" (p. 130). Curtis' auditory skills improved as he followed along in the text when it was my turn to read. My reading, as well as his own, exposed him to a volume of language beyond the level of ordinary conversation. Reading back and forth made it easy and natural to uncover gaps in understanding and fill them in.

Collaborative reading advanced Curtis' reading competence in several important ways. It whetted Curtis' appetite for reading and provided a model of skillful oral reading (Anderson et al. 1985). The questions and discussion that arose during this and subsequent reading experiences helped him integrate what he was reading with what he already knew. This ability characterizes good readers of every age (Bransford et al. 1982).

In discussing the problems of early readers, Beck et al. (1981) state that "each interaction with text should reinforce the notion that reading is a process through which meaning is gathered" (p. 780). Curtis' reading, at first halting and uncertain, slowly became more confident and expressive. Our oral reading, along with the dialogue it engendered, helped bring *The Chalkbox Kid* to life and imbue it with meaning.

As the number of books read in this way increased, associations between ideas, characters, and themes arose in the same conversational tone. All the elements of reading comprehension were there, but in a way that felt natural and spontaneous rather than pedantic.

As language and reading develop, children need to attain the speed and fluency essential to reading with comprehension. Carbo (1997) offers a continuum of methods of reading to and with children that bring children closer to this goal. Carbo's modeling methods are to be used with material that is within children's language levels and just beyond their independent reading levels.

In contrast, the "My Turn-Your Turn" approach is particularly suited to developing the language that makes reading meaningful. Reading collaboratively provides opportunities to pause and clarify unfamiliar vocabulary, grammar, and syntax. This makes it possible to read with children at the limit of their language and comprehension levels.

Educational researcher Frank Smith (1985) affirms the value of collaborative reading:

> It is important to read to children, but even more important to read *with* them. Children get their first chance to solve many of the problems of reading when they and adults are reading the same text at the same time (p. 134).

Smith observes that once children develop a little proficiency in reading, their eyes move ahead of the teacher's voice. They begin to read independent of adult assistance. As competence and confidence develop, children tend to pull ahead of the adult until eventually they are able to manage alone.

My own experience bears this out. With almost every child, the first chapter book has taken a long time to get through and has required constant supervision and encouragement. Little by little, the struggle lessens. A sense of ease creeps into the children's reading. Children need to get their fill of listening and reading at this level so they can move as smoothly and confidently as possible into the next.

Chapter 9

Reading for Self-Discovery

"Education means this: to be learning what is your own, and what is not your own."

Epictetus

Curtis' reading of *The Chalkbox Kid* evolved into an approach that has opened up the world of reading to children of all levels. Collaborative reading has given even the youngest and least experienced readers access to stories that would otherwise have been beyond their ability to understand and appreciate. Some of these have engendered strong feelings of connection between book and reader.

The following stories are among those that have had particular meaning to individual children. They encompass both fiction and nonfiction. Most of the books were read by children age nine and older. Some were semi-independent readers, while others could barely read unassisted. Because all the children had a long way to go in reading, nearly all these books were read jointly in the resource room.

FICTION: A SAMPLING

Roderick the Red (McCullagh 1958)

John had spent five years in school with an unidentified hearing loss. He entered the resource room program as a fourth grader with fair oral language, but little sight vocabulary and no word attack skills. Somehow, John's enthusiasm for reading had survived undiminished. *Roderick the Red*, a pirate story with controlled vocabulary and repetitive language patterns, was just the book for this ten-year-old beginning reader. John was caught up in the suspense and adventure of a fearsome pirate roaming the high seas in search of his sack of gold. He borrowed the book to reread with his father, and did not relinquish it for several months.

Brown Beauty (Webster 1968)

Numerous children have been moved by this story of a faithful farm horse and the boy who did not want to see her replaced by a tractor. On the way to the market to be sold, the horse saves the farmer's life as the tractor begins to careen down an icy hill. Over and over, children's compassion has been aroused by the plight of Brown Beauty, who could be a friend and was capable of thinking for herself in a way that the tractor could not.

Sally the Seagull (Webster 1968)

This book by the author of *Brown Beauty* tells the story of a seagull saved by a sailor. The seagull, in turn, saves Jim's fishing boat from going down in a storm. The life-and-death drama of both plot and illustrations have kept beginning readers of all ages on the edge of their seats.

Mortimer (Munsch 1985)

Clang, clang, rattle-bing-bang
Gonna make my noise all day.
Clang, clang, rattle-bing-bang
Gonna make my noise all day.

Mortimer's mother, father, seventeen brothers and sisters, and two policemen all take turns thump-thump-thumping up the stairs and telling Mortimer to "BE QUIET!" Mortimer nods his head "yes" each time, and bursts into song the moment he hears the last footstep die away. Mortimer's timid yet exuberant defiance as portrayed by both story and illustrations have made this the all-time favorite book of younger children. Nancy, a severely hard-of-hearing kindergarten child with a late start in developing language, memorized the refrain, which she belted out at every opportunity.

The Legend of the Bluebonnet (dePaola 1983)

The appeal of picture books reaches beyond the earliest grades. In this story, a young girl orphaned by famine creeps out of her tipi to sacrifice her doll to the Great Spirits. The drought ends, and She-Who-Is-Alone becomes known as "One-Who-Dearly-Loved-Her-People." Curtis, at age eleven, responded to the beauty and simplicity of Tomi de Paola's language and illustrations.

The Spider, the Cave and the Pottery Bowl (Clymer 1971)

Shortly after falling in love with *The Legend of the Blue-bonnet*, Curtis discovered this short novel. In it, two Indian children find the special clay their grandmother needs to make her famous pottery. Curtis was able to read this book on his own with enough ease to experience the grandmother's sorrow at having run out of clay, the children's adventures in finding it, and the family's quiet satisfaction in making pottery together once again.

The Bears' House (Sachs 1971)

This is the story of a ten-year-old girl whose mother is incapacitated by depression, and whose siblings are raising themselves. At every opportunity, Fran Ellen retreats into fantasy in front of the miniature bears' house in the corner of the classroom. This was the first chapter book ever read independently by Cynthia, an eleven-year-old fifth grader with a severe hearing loss. Cynthia grasped both the story line and the nuances of the character portrayals, and related the story to me with a good deal of feeling.

The Chocolate Touch (Catling 1988)

Cynthia, Shelley, Crystal, and Tom selected this book from the spring book fair. I hoped it would serve as a shot-in-the-arm to keep the last few weeks of school alive to the end. Every day I passed around a different chocolate treat before beginning to read. After eating our way through tootsie rolls, tootsie pops, and Hershey kisses Cynthia suddenly exclaimed, "Oh, now I get it why you give us chocolate every day!" Humor and drama moved us along in spite of some difficult language, and the book was a huge success.

Sideways Stories from Wayside School (Sachar 1985)

Twenty-eight children and two teachers, one of whom wiggles her ears and turns children into apples, each rate a short chapter in this hilarious book. The individual sketches are loosely connected, and can be read in random order. The book became a collective resource room undertaking. We drew a building with thirty classroom windows. Whenever a child had a few extra minutes, he or she would select and read a chapter and write the number of that chapter on the corresponding window (see p. 80). Getting through the book stretched over several months, since we fitted it in around other work and there was no pressure to complete it. The children enjoyed beating one another to chapters they particularly wanted to read. Each chapter was funnier and sillier than the one before.

NONFICTION: A SAMPLING

Outside-In (Smallman 1986)

Every child has contributed to the dog-eared condition of this clear and informative book about the human body. Two-page spreads give simple descriptions of such topics as "Breathing," "Bones and Teeth," and "What Happens to Your Food?" Younger children are content with the figures of boys and girls, clothed and unclothed. Flaps lift up to reveal bones, muscle, intestines, etc.

The Glorious Flight (Provensen 1987)

This Caldecott Medal winner is a witty account of the first flight across the English Channel in 1909. Tom selected this book when he was in sixth grade because he loved biographies and science. Much of the language was beyond him. Reading with and to him, paraphrasing some sections and omitting others, brought the story within his grasp. Tom's love of history and science, enhanced by his sense of humor, made this book a vivid one for him.

Albert Einstein (Lepscky 1982)

About one hundred years ago, there lived a boy named
  Albert Einstein.
Albert was a strange boy.
Always absent-minded.
Always messy.
It was a difficult job for him to tie his shoes.

Furthermore, Albert hated history and geography, seldom joined the other children in their games, yet never stopped asking questions about the universe. The reader was a ten-year-old boy with a newly diagnosed hearing loss. John's academic skills were minimal, and he walked around in a state of constant puzzlement. At the same time, he had an active and inquiring mind and a love of science. This book struck a chord in him.

Marco Polo: His Notebook (Roth 1990)

This work of historical fiction in diary form is based on Marco Polo's notebooks. The pages have the look of parchment, with handsome woodcuts and engravings. The entries are short, and give a taste of each leg of Marco Polo's journey. Curtis, reading this book in sixth grade, had a rich imagination and some sense of history and geography. For him the book was a compelling eye-opener to exotic times and places.

How Much Is A Million? (Schwarz 1985)

"If one million kids climbed onto one another's shoulders, they would be . . . higher than the highest mountains." This book came close to becoming the private property of a third-grade boy struggling to learn English, but who loved and excelled in math. Tom read and reread it from third grade all the way through sixth. The enormity of millions, billions, and trillions kept drawing him back to this humorously illustrated book, which attempts to make astronomical numbers comprehensible by relating them to familiar concepts.

The Microscope (Kumin 1986)

Arnold Lobel's pen and ink drawings portray Anton van Leeuwenhoek's invention of the microscope with humor and scientific accuracy. This synopsis in verse form of his great achievement was thoroughly enjoyed by Crystal, Shelley, and Curtis when they were in fifth grade. It served as an introduction to the concept and spirit of the Renaissance.

Go Free or Die: A Story about Harriet Tubman (Ferris 1988)

Harriet Tubman's life is simply and powerfully portrayed in four chapters and an epilogue, with clear print and memorable full-page illustrations throughout. Three children have been deeply impressed by this book. Eleven-year-old Tom was absorbed by the events as he followed them on the map provided in the back of the book. At the same age, Crystal expressed her understanding in a book report that ended: "Harriet was a slave woman who wanted her people free and her self [*sic*] too. Time after time she brought her people up north to freedom. She took a chance that she might die. She risked her life to help her people."

Douglas, in second grade, had surprised me by asking searching questions about the life of Dr. Martin Luther King, Jr. This led us to attempt reading *Go Free Or Die*. Douglas' relevant and astute observations showed that the book was within his grasp, and an important source of learning for him.

Keep the Lights Burning, Abbie (Roop 1985)

This beginning-to-read portrayal of an actual happening made a page from history accessible to Crystal and Curtis, two eleven-year-olds who were about the same age as the heroine of the story. Abbie overcomes her fears and takes on the responsibility of climbing the lighthouse stairs one stormy week to make sure the lights are burning while her father is away. The children who read the book had passed the "easy-to-read" stage, and were reading fiction on a much higher level. But the world of nonfiction reading was new to them, and it felt logical to take a step back and start over with easier reading material. Books such as this one appealed to the children, and freed them to concentrate on the concepts and information without having to struggle with the reading itself.

The Titanic: Lost . . . and Found (Donnelly 1987)

Tom and Curtis, two boys who gravitated toward nonfiction, were engrossed by this saga of the Titanic. The story is a Step-Into-Reading book published by Random House. Sentence structure is kept simple, with informative illustrations on every page.

Witch Hunt: It Happened in Salem Village (Krensky 1989)

Curtis and Cynthia, both fifth graders, were incredulous as we read this book together. They could hardly wait to pick up where we had left off the day before. The vocabulary and language concepts of this Random House Step-Into-Reading book were way beyond them. But as stumbling blocks were cleared away, the children's fascination with the content carried them along.

Living in Prehistoric Times (Chisholm 1982)

This is the first in a series of "Usborne First History" books, which introduce children to major historical periods. The illustrations are vivid and dramatic. In addition to the main text, bubbles are used to highlight and explain details of the pictures. The book is dense with information. John and Cathy, two ten-year olds with little general knowledge, loved making their way through parts of the book as we read and discussed each new concept. Though slow and painstaking, the time was well spent. Every concept they acquired (e.g., hunting, weaving, shelter) laid a foundation for understanding development through the ages.

READING: A DEEPER SIGNIFICANCE

Books are more than steppingstones to higher reading scores. Children who live with a rich assortment of reading material appropriate to their reading levels and interests discover books that come to have deep personal relevance. A book that captivates one child may be of little interest to another. No reading list or guiding hand can predict these connections, which are as varied as the children's personalities, backgrounds, and inclinations.

Each book described above, among others, kindled a spark in the child or children who read it. My feeling has been that the spark is one of self-recognition, in the sense of an encounter with something deeply meaningful that resonates in the reader. It is as if such an encounter gives the child a piece of who he or she is. A moment like this is deeply moving. It is the essence of education.

Chapter 10

Reading Aloud

As the children's competence in reading gradually increased, I continued reading to them. I selected books beyond their independent reading level that could enrich their language and listening skills. My acquaintance with children's literature had been limited to books suitable for young deaf children just beginning to develop language. That meant a relatively small body of books having clear, simple pictures that conveyed the whole story, a few carefully chosen words, and repetitive refrains. The "Treasury" of Jim Trelease's *Read-Aloud Handbook* (1985) served as a starting point for an organized and systematic exploration of children's literature.

SPRINGBOARD TO LANGUAGE

For most young children, the language of every-day life provides the foundation from which early reading grows. Reading, in turn, sparks growth in language, and a spiral of reading-language development has begun.

In discussing the close tie between reading and language, Butler and Clay (1979) maintain:

It is certain that listening to stories expands the vocabulary. The speech of children who are used to "book language" is often rich and varied. This is easy to understand; such children have a large stock of words and ideas to draw on. This stock just has to help when they are later trying to make sense of a line of print. They need resources to call on, then.

How can a beginning reader, groping for a word, find it unless it is in his or her mind to begin with? (p. 20)

Reading aloud is invaluable in creating the language foundation that many deaf and hard-of-hearing children lack. As with all children, reading aloud can continue to spur language development long after basic competence has been attained.

Emily and Sarah: Two Little Girls

In his outline of read-aloud stages, Trelease cites *The Courage of Sarah Noble* (Dalgliesh 1954) as an example of a longer, but still beginning, chapter book. It is the story of a young girl in colonial times who accompanies her father on his journey to find a new home for their family. I wondered whether Sarah's feelings and experiences might appeal to Emily, who was approximately the same age.

Emily displayed characteristics of a language disorder unrelated to her mild to moderate hearing loss. These included idiosyncrasies in oral language, along with difficulty responding to questions and relating a story or experience. It soon became apparent that Emily's pleasure in listening to the story was accompanied by deficits in comprehension.

From Abstract to Concrete

In order to bolster Emily's understanding of the story by making Sarah's journey come alive, I employed a combination of strategies. One was acting out key incidents. Another was relating what we had read as storytelling partners.

Once they had reached their destination, Sarah's father built his daughter a bed of logs. Emily and I took an imaginary walk in the woods. We drew an ax and cut it out. We pantomimed chopping down trees and sawing them into logs. We talked about what it must feel like to lie on a bed made of rough logs. We reread the chapter with new understanding.

Co-Telling the Story

The next morning, I asked Emily to tell me a little about what we had read the day before. Nothing came to her mind. Reminding her of our walk in the woods refreshed Emily's memory and helped her recall parts of the sequence leading to the bed of logs.

Retelling the story together enabled Emily to visualize missing details. I would begin by relating a scene. A sentence or two usually sparked her memory. When this happened, she would interrupt with excitement. The story was now in her hands. Emily would move the story forward a few sentences, occasionally even longer, before losing the thread. I would pick up as she left off until Emily again found her way back into the story.

Norris and Damico (1990) emphasize the importance of employing holistic language teaching with language-disordered children. They observe that working on word order and pronouns won't help children learn to tell a story, whereas engaging in storytelling will help children learn to use word order and pronouns. For Emily, co-telling the journey and adventures of Sarah Noble provided the opportunity to strengthen semi-familiar language concepts and acquire new ones.

Reading *The Courage of Sarah Noble* showed me what Emily could understand, given a great deal of support and guidance. It seemed likely that she would bring those same needs to another book of comparable difficulty. I sensed that, for Emily, moving "ahead" meant going back to the fairy tales and picture books of earliest childhood. At this point, these would meet her emotional and language-learning needs in ways that more demanding beginning chapter books could not.

Emily's mother provided support in immersing her daughter in this kind of reading at home, in addition to the reading we were doing at school. It was not quite a year later when Emily produced her first page-long piece of writing: a fluent, well-shaped story about a ghost-man who lived "deep, deep in the forest." This landmark attested to the beginnings of literacy in a little girl who was gaining the foundation she needed to move forward, at her own pace, as a reader and writer.

It had taken a long time to find the key that would open the door to reading for children with profound language deficits due to hearing loss. Unlike Emily, with her specific language disorder, a number of children were moving along with increasing ease and independence from one beginning chapter book to another. Longer chapter books, once an impossible dream, were almost within reach. I pictured the children reading with abandon, ready to partake of the worlds that awaited them in the finest of children's literature. Adventure and reflection, sorrow and humor—all would be richly available to them as it was to other young readers. Reading aloud helped pave the way to this goal.

OUR FIRST CHAPTER BOOK

Many pressing needs clamor to be addressed in the short resource room period. It is difficult to brush them aside in order to devote session after session to the sustained reading of a lengthy book. But, as different children have stood on the threshold of attempting their first "real" chapter book, I felt that it was important to do exactly that.

Three fifth graders arrived at this point at more or less the same time. A disheveled red-headed mischief maker swept us, bubbling with laughter and excitement, into the realm of her adventures. Our weeks spent in the company of Pippi Longstocking (Lindgren 1970) on her roller coaster of escapades was a memorable interlude in resource room life.

Many a children's novel could have served as an introduction to this genre of writing. I chose *Pippi Longstocking* for the following reasons.

- My memory of having discovered the book as an adult was still fresh, and I was eager to pass that experience along to the children.
- The story is rooted in the familiar and moves on from there. The everyday life of a nine-year-old girl would serve as a basis for listening with comprehension.
- That Pippi lives on her own with a horse and a monkey for company, refuses to go to school, and is shockingly and delightfully irreverent in every way would provide ample scope for imagination and humor.
- The language of the book was straightforward enough for the children to comprehend with relative ease: "[Pippi's] hair, the color of a carrot, was braided in two tight braids that stuck straight out. Her nose was the shape of a very small potato and was dotted all over with freckles." At the same time, unfamiliar words, idioms, and sentence structures would extend the children's vocabulary and language.

Integrating Language

Pippi Longstocking offered abundant opportunities to integrate language and reading. Enticing vocabulary and idioms, along with higher levels of grammar and syntax, awaited us on every page: "Tommy and Annika . . . were so utterly absorbed in the story"; "As it was raining cats and dogs . . ."; "I wonder what you would have said if I had come along. . . ."

I did not attempt to teach new vocabulary in any formal way. Instead, I explained unfamiliar words and concepts casually and moved on, as one might with any child. I realized that the children had enough of a language foundation to begin to acquire language in this way.

I wanted to make sure that unfamiliar vocabulary and language concepts did not hinder the children's full enjoyment of the story. As frequently as needed, I offered running "simultaneous translations" into more familiar language, then restored the word to its original context:

"A remarkable child," said one of the sailors . . .

Remarkable means "amazing": an amazing child—a remarkable child.

"Is this the girl who has moved into Villa Villekula?" asked one of the policemen. "Certainly not," said Pippi. "Quite the contrary."

Contrary means "opposite": "Not me," said Pippi. "Quite the contrary."

As we went along, I was alert to the children's reactions. Exclamations of surprise, hilarity, or disbelief confirmed their understanding of what was happening in the story. We took these opportunities to laugh together and share our responses before moving on.

An absence of reaction to humorous incidents signaled a lack of comprehension. The stumbling block usually turned out to be an unfamiliar word, or an allusion to a part of the world that was outside the children's experience. I kept explanations as brief as possible so as not to interrupt the flow of the story.

Reading aloud introduced a level of language that the children had not experienced in ordinary conversation: "After the policemen had stood there a while wondering what to do, they went and got a ladder, lined it against one of the gables of the house, and then climbed up, first one policeman and then the other, to get Pippi down." Although difficult at first, the children became accustomed to the lengthy and complex sentences as we went along.

"My name is Pippilotta Delicatessa Windowshade Mackrel-mint Efraim's Daughter Longstocking. . . ." At an age when other very young children delight in whimsy, children with hearing impairments are likely to be struggling with the language of the "here and now." At age eleven, with a solid grounding in every-day language, the children were able to savor the fantastic, the ridiculous, the absurd moments in *Pippi Longstocking*.

Ongoing discussion, sometimes guided and sometimes spontaneous, provided opportunities for children to express their reactions to the events of the story. If conveying a thought became too cumbersome, I intervened: "What Shelley is saying is. . . ." This helped children past difficulties with the mechanics of language, and communicated respect for the content of what they were trying to say.

BRINGING STORIES TO LIFE

Activities that accompany a read-aloud can be effective in helping children orient their listening and sustain focus. These activities need to reflect the spirit of the book. They need to keep enthusiasm high and clarify aspects of the story that are essential to comprehension, while remaining secondary to the story itself.

Activities can take many forms. Picking a chapter and fill-ing in that number on a window kept the children's eagerness from flagging as we read randomly selected chapters from *Sideways Stories from the Wayside School* (Sachar 1985):

Using chalk on black paper to design a garden enhanced several children's appreciation of the garden created by Gregory in *The Chalkbox Kid* (Bulla 1987) on the walls of a burned-out building:

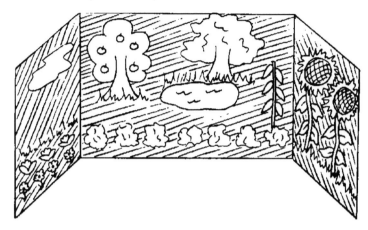

Role playing, with props, had helped Emily grasp the highlights of Sarah Noble's journey. Two activities clarified aspects of *Pippi Longstocking* that otherwise would have remained elusive. A sheet entitled "Tall Tales" provided a focus for the children's listening: "In Egypt, everybody walks backwards! People walk on their hands in India! Not a single person in the Belgian Congo tells the truth! In Brazil, everybody goes around with egg in their hair! In Guatemala, people sleep with their feet on the pillow and their heads under the quilt! It's against the law for children to have lessons in Argentina!"

Writing came into play as children identified whopper after whopper in their reading and added them to the list. At the same time, children colored in each country on an outline map of the world, which sparkled with the locations of Pippi's far-flung adventures.

Best of all was our convivial hilarity during those weeks of reading. "Pluttification" struck a tragicomic chord in three children whose grasp of math was tenuous in the extreme. Many humorous allusions lived on in the resource room community long after Pippi's adventures had come to an end.

ON THE HORIZON

Pippi Longstocking led the way to the semi-independent and, eventually, independent reading of innumerable chapter books. In Trelease's outline of reading stages (1985), chapter books are followed by full-length novels. In these, description enriches the development of plot, character, and setting. Trelease notes that experienced listeners may have the attention span and imagination to be ready for a full length novel by kindergarten.

Few deaf and hard-of-hearing kindergarten children have come this far in their language development. In sixth grade, Curtis gleaned enough from his reading of *Where the Red Fern Grows* (Rawls 1974) to be moved by the story. But even combined classroom and resource room exposure could not bring the language of the book comfortably within his grasp.

In my memory is a picture of Curtis, a newly transplanted first grader, with few sight words and no phonics concepts. He lacked the vocabulary to communicate what he liked to eat, to play, to draw. He was at a loss to understand and enjoy the simplest of picture books until adapted to his language level.

As time went on, Curtis' love affair with books sustained him in the slow process of gaining competence as a reader. There is reason to trust that, one day, Curtis' reading will grow to encompass the full-length novels now beyond his reach.

Reading together in the resource room led to a variety of activities designed to teach specific skills. Of these, vocabulary development was of paramount importance.

Chapter 11

Building Vocabulary

"Ms. Stelling, would you carry my bookbag?" asked ten-year-old Curtis one day at the top of the staircase. "How come?" I wondered, forgetting that he had not been feeling well that morning. "My head feels like the solar system going around," Curtis responded. Once downstairs, he elaborated, "I feel like the king of tornadoes."

Three years earlier, Curtis had barely been able to engage in conversation or respond to simple questions. His knowledge of English had grown painfully slowly for what seemed like a long time. I questioned whether Curtis was impaired in his ability to acquire language, or whether this rate of progress was to be expected of a hard-of-hearing child with little exposure to English outside of school.

The experience of reading *The Chalkbox Kid* marked a turning point in Curtis' comprehension and ability to express himself. His rate of language acquisition gradually accelerated until, one day, Curtis had at his command the words he needed to communicate his experience of the world in vivid and colorful language.

FACTORS IN VOCABULARY ACQUISITION

In introducing a study of the vocabulary development of preschool children, Bloom describes children who began to acquire words "with a learning trajectory that took off like a small rocket" while others "were much slower to get off the ground, and their trajectories were forever in the shadow of the other children" (Hart and Risley 1995, x).

Incorporating weekly field trips in the children's school experience did not result in the acceleration of vocabulary growth. Relating each new experience to what children already knew by means of small-group discussions before and after each trip, with opportunities for role play, resulted in a "spurt of new vocabulary words" and an "abrupt acceleration in [children's] vocabulary growth curves" (p. 15). Yet the increases did not continue beyond the immediate activity. Hart and Risley concluded that "We found we could easily increase the size of children's vocabularies by teaching them new words. But we could not accelerate the rate of vocabulary growth so that it would continue beyond direct teaching; we could not change the developmental trajectory."

Two factors correlated with differences in vocabulary development. The first was the variety of experiences in a child's life, as reflected in the range and volume of words used by parents. The authors found that "the more often a child hears words used in association with a variety of events and other words, the more varied and refined are the meanings of words for the child" (p. 150).

The second factor was the ratio of encouragement to discouragement with regard to language usage. Discouragement took the form of prohibitions ("Quit it." "You better not . . .") without the substitution of acceptable alternatives. Language growth was also inhibited when parents did not repeat or expand on children's utterances. In contrast, three-year olds with extensive vocabularies had received "three years of being told that they were 'right' and 'good,' and three years of frequently being chosen as more interesting to listen to and talk to than anyone else" (p. 183).

TWO PATHS TO WORD KNOWLEDGE

For children who are deaf and hard of hearing, as for all children, having a limited vocabulary "limits both comprehension and expression, restricting and confining the possible use of one's powers" (O'Connor 1964). Words are the building blocks of language. As such, vocabulary development has occupied a place of unrivaled importance in the resource room period.

Anderson and Nagy (1992) argue that typical definition-based vocabulary-building programs are not effective in increasing comprehension and word usage. My own experience

corroborates that an assortment of drills based on randomly selected words of the week does not necessarily bring those
words into a child's active or even passive vocabulary.

The clearest of definitions is likely to contain words that
are themselves unfamiliar to children who are deaf and hard of
hearing. Often a child needs to understand a whole network of
concepts in order to grasp the meaning of a word. A dictionary
or glossary cannot lay the groundwork by drawing on the
child's own knowledge and experience and moving on from
there to illuminate word meaning and usage:

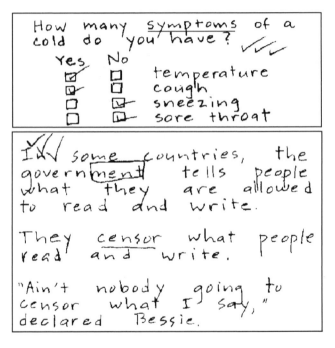

Anderson and Nagy suggest a more promising possibility.
They point to studies indicating that children who do a fair
amount of independent reading can easily acquire thousands of
words a year as the incidental by-product of reading. Deaf and
hard-of-hearing children are likely to need more direct instruction. Even then, they rarely have the language foundation to gain
new words at anything approaching this rate. Yet for them, as for
all children, reading offers a joyful and optimistic alternative to
memorizing word lists as a source of vocabulary development.

VOCABULARY CARDS

Means to an End

No aspect of the resource room experience engenders more anticipation or satisfaction than vocabulary expansion that grows out of reading and conversing together.

Over the years I have found a way of working on word recognition and comprehension that has resulted in vocabulary increases of as much as six hundred words in one year. This is very little compared with the thousands of new words children normally learn each year. What feels hopeful is that the children are gaining a grounding in word knowledge that may gradually make incidental learning possible.

Expanding vocabulary as described below is a structured approach to developing a specific skill. When integrated into a full range of receptive and expressive language activities, it becomes an important facet of a natural language program.

I keep on hand a large supply of strips cut from 12" x 18" construction paper.

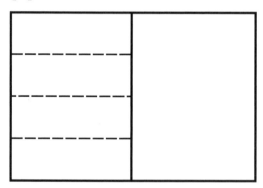

Younger children enjoy the colors and easy-to-handle size of the construction paper; older children may appreciate graduating to index cards. Any dark marker, not necessarily black, is good for printing words.

As we begin to read, it is not long before a child misreads or stumbles over a word. We pause. I print the word or phrase on a card. I give the child whatever explanation is necessary regarding the meaning of an unfamiliar word, or the phonics needed to sound out a word that is known but not recognized. The words are put into an envelope marked "Words" or "Vocabulary."

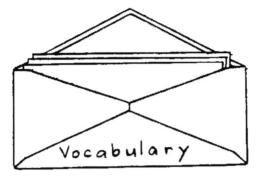

Children take their envelopes home in their home-school notebooks with reminders to parents to go over vocabulary that evening (* = "homework").

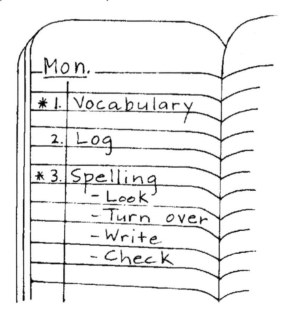

Listening to children read their words is undemanding and minimally time-consuming. Many parents who have difficulty assisting with other learning tasks do listen regularly as their children review their words. This daily reinforcement makes all the difference. When no parent is available, the child is left to practice unfamiliar words on his or her own. This is far from ideal. Depending on the child's reading and/or language level, it may be altogether unrealistic, and expectations need to be adjusted accordingly.

Adopting and Adapting

The use of vocabulary cards has been adapted from the work of two educators: Fernald (1943) and Ashton-Warner (1963).

Fernald employed a multi-kinesthetic approach to teaching dyslexic children. She excerpted misspelled words from children's own compositions and wrote them in crayon on cards. Children read their words as they traced the waxy letters with their fingers. The words were reviewed in subsequent sessions. As children read, they gave each word a check in the corner. Words with three checks were filed in shoeboxes in alphabetical order.

With a stack of blank cards and a big black crayon, Ashton-Warner elicited from children words that vividly expressed their feelings and experiences. Children practiced reading their words to one another. Spelling and writing evolved from their vocabulary, which became the key to literacy for these children.

> "Mohi," I ask a new five, an undisciplined Maori.
> "What do you want?"
> "Jet!"
> I smile and write it on a strong little card and give it to him.
> "What is it again?"
> "Jet!"
> "You can bring it back in the morning. What do you want, Gay?"
> Gay is the classic overdisciplined, bullied victim of the respectable mother.
> "House," she whispers. So I write that, too, and give it into her eager hand.
> "What do you want, Seven?" Seven is a violent Maori.
> "Bomb! Bomb! I want bomb!"
> So Seven gets his word "bomb" and challenges anyone to take it away from him (pp. 35–36).

The needs and abilities of deaf and hard-of-hearing children differ in several respects from those of the children described above. Unlike dyslexic children, children with hearing impairments typically do not require a multi-kinesthetic approach to learning to read. The group dynamics vital to Ashton-Warner's work cannot easily be carried over into the one-to-one or small group resource room setting.

Most young children with hearing impairments have yet to acquire the language facility that served as the basis for the work of these two teachers. Ashton-Warner's children had words at their command, but needed to learn to read them. Fernald's children had words at their command, but needed to learn to spell them. With children who are deaf and hard of hearing, vocabulary cards have served to develop language at a more basic level.

Used toward this end, word cards have become a means of introducing not only words, but phrases, sentence patterns, synonyms, antonyms, grammar, and syntax. Science, social studies, children's literature, and casual conversation have all become rich sources of language for vocabulary cards.

Other aspects of Fernald's and Ashton-Warner's methods have lent themselves to being adopted as is into the resource room curriculum. Vocabulary cards, along with Fernald's method of checking words as they are reviewed and filing those that have been mastered, provide a clear and appealing format for systematic vocabulary expansion. Using children's own interests and experiences as the basis for language development is well suited to the needs of young deaf and hard-of-hearing children.

Categories

These apparently simple word cards can be made to serve a variety of underlying purposes.

Reinforcing new words or phrases:

tow truck	Niagara Falls

Expanding vocabulary through synonyms:

a row of . . . a series of . . .	That dog is harmless. He won't hurt you.

Expanding vocabulary through opposites:

Opposites:
    a lot
    a few
	Opposites:
	 Take a book.
	 Replace the book.

Building on a familiar word:

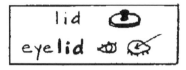

Illustrating word usage:

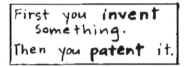

Developing awareness of tense:

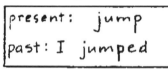

Clarifying formation of plurals:

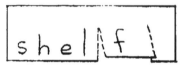

Developing understanding of contractions:

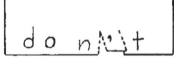

Reinforcing phonics rules:

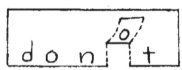

Refining word discrimination:

invite
invent

carve
cover

"The Rich Get Richer"

Vocabulary knowledge facilitates reading comprehension; reading further expands vocabulary; this leads, in turn, to more efficient reading. Stanovich (1986) refers to this spiral as the "Matthew Effect in Reading" (p. 380).

While "the rich"—children who read well and have good vocabularies—"get richer," children with inadequate vocabularies read less, and with less enjoyment. As a result, their vocabularies grow more slowly, further inhibiting growth in reading.

Breaking this cycle is one of the imperatives of resource room teaching. Vocabulary cards have helped make this possible.

SHARED READING: BRIDGE TO VOCABULARY DEVELOPMENT

The language recorded on word cards comes from a variety of sources. Chief among them is literature. Carbo (1987) confirms my experience that youngsters with reading difficulties recall words presented in the context of a well-written story more rapidly than words in isolation or words presented in poorly conceived or poorly written stories. Children quickly become accustomed to moving from a story to the making of a vocabulary card and back again. We may continue where we left off, or reread the sentence from which the word was taken, this time with full understanding.

At age eight, Robert seemed to have a fair amount of language. Reading together exposed the fact that, in spite of having only a mild to moderate hearing loss, Robert could not use the words he knew to respond accurately to questions or to relate specific incidents. This held true for ordinary conversation as well. When asked how he had enjoyed spending time with his uncle over the weekend, Robert replied: "What uncle you mean—there's two different kinds of uncle. Oh, you mean the aunt one."

It took many guided discussions before Robert began to respond with some degree of accuracy to questions generated by *Dan Frontier* (Hurley 1966), an early reading book about pioneer days. Excerpting words and expanding on them provided a format for language development. Even familiar words opened the door to new concepts and to the language needed to convey them.

```
house
cabin
log cabin
```

The familiar word "house" led to a discussion of what cabins, then chimneys, were made of. It took Robert several days to grasp that chimneys, unlike cabins, had to be built of stone. It took several days longer before he could formulate his understanding in one or two simple sentences. Slowly Robert became better able to mobilize his thoughts and express them in connected language triggered by the words and phrases on the vocabulary cards.

In contrast, Curtis' comprehension of what he read was basically sound. But his vocabulary was limited, and he frequently encountered words he did not know. This hampered his understanding of the story.

Word cards brought meaning to Curtis' reading of *The Chalkbox Kid*, his earliest chapter book. In addition to expanding vocabulary, the cards offered opportunities for checking comprehension as we progressed through the story.

A passage from *The Chalkbox Kid* describes Gregory drawing his garden in chalk on the walls of a burned-out building. He rubbed out a ship and an alligator; they didn't belong in the garden. He made rows of vegetables, then added sunflowers and poles with sweet peas on them. Gregory drew a path leading to a pool, and put a toad by the pool.

By moving from familiar to unfamiliar concepts, vocabulary cards clarified unfamiliar language, and helped Curtis make his way through a difficult book.

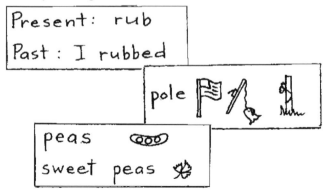

VOCABULARY AND NONFICTION READING

Experience stories had introduced Douglas to reading in kindergarten. Two years later, Douglas' interests, and his reading, had begun to branch out in the direction of science and history.

Douglas had no background information or vocabulary related to any area of science when he became fascinated by bats and space in mid-second grade. Word cards helped crystallize the many concepts presented in *The Earth and the Sky* (Gallimard and Verdet 1989). They enabled Douglas to absorb this information so thoroughly that he was well prepared for further reading on this topic.

As we progressed through the book, I began leaving blank spaces, with the missing information written on the backs of the cards. This gave Douglas a chance to exercise his memory. I wondered whether he would find this frustrating. Instead, Douglas rose to the challenge of memorizing the planets and other information related to space and geography. He experienced a moment of satisfaction each time he turned a card over and found his answer validated.

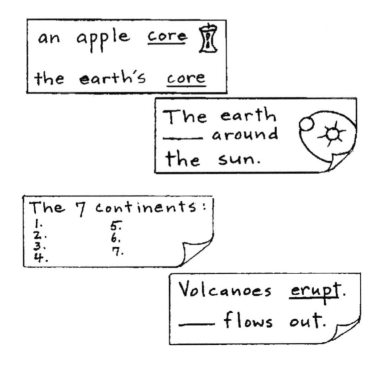

The earth ○
_____ on its
axis.

The _____ is the
coldest place
on earth.

The E_____ is
the hottest part
of the earth.

The first astro-
naut to walk on
the moon was _____

The planet with
rings around it
is _____.

The closest planet
to the sun is _____.
The farthest is
_____.

The temperature
on _____ is just
right for living
things.

○ full moon
☽ crescent moon

Touching on every card three days in a row afforded Douglas opportunities to do his own thinking. He wondered how planets stay up in space, and what makes them orbit. He prepared a diagram of the solar system to present to his science teacher in the hope that she could satisfy his curiosity. For this highly intelligent eight-year-old, simple cards conceived to expand vocabulary proved to be mind-expanding as well.

A system that had helped introduce Douglas to science became valuable in another area of nonfiction reading. Soon after reading *The Earth and the Sky*, Douglas requested a book about Martin Luther King. We located a two-page spread in *One-Minute Stories of Great Americans* (Lewis 1990). This account of Dr. King's life contained words and ideas that were new to Douglas. I suspected that concepts such as segregation, integration, and civil rights would be somewhat beyond his ability to grasp, and would not sustain his interest.

I underestimated Douglas. His questions and observations were insightful and to the point. Our reading of this mini-biography, which took several days, suggested two new uses of vocabulary cards. The first was assembling cards into vocabulary booklets; the second was using songs to enhance vocabulary and language.

NEW POSSIBILITIES

In reading with a child, I pick and choose which words to put on cards and which to pass over so as not to lose the child's interest. Martin Luther King's life generated many important words and concepts, all of which called for clarification. This would take thought on my part. Not wanting Douglas' interest to flag, I put off making word cards until after our session was over. I wondered whether they would seem distant and removed when I brought them out the next day. This was not the case.

Dr. Martin Luther King, Jr. was a leader in the Civil Rights Movement.

T.: "Hey, give me the ball!"

G.: "I have a right to play with it."

People have the right to get a drink from any water fountain.

It's a civil right.

M.L.K. didn't want people to be violent.

He wanted people to be non-violent.

How did Black people fight for their civil rights? Not with fists. Not with guns. They had...

We want our civil rights.

... peaceful demonstrations.

Black children and white children were segregated.

M. L. King wanted child-
ren to be <u>integrated</u>.

M.L. King said:
"<u>I have a dream</u> that
some day all people
will be equal."

M.L. King was
<u>assassinated</u>.

We <u>honor</u> Dr. Mar-
tin Luther King, Jr.

As we related the story of Dr. King's life using the vocabulary cards, it occurred to me to staple them together into a
booklet. Creating a new and distinctive format proved successful in several ways. First, it kept the vocabulary cards together
in a coherent sequence. Second, it elevated this chapter in history to the status it deserved. Most importantly, it endowed an
abstract historical event with meaning and relevance.
Subsequent vocabulary booklets have achieved similar results.

The last thing I extracted from the biography of Martin
Luther King was the opening stanza of "We Shall Overcome."
Douglas, a thorough child, insisted on all four stanzas. These
formed a separate vocabulary book. Douglas loved singing all
of the verses every day. He was not willing to set the book aside

once it had received its three checks. We sang the Freedom Song
every morning for weeks, and at intervals after that.

Although carrying a tune is out of the question because of
his hearing loss, Douglas improved in being able to sing the
words in rhythm, which had also been difficult for him. This
made singing a valuable exercise in auditory training.

I believe that Douglas would not have been as drawn to
this song had it not conveyed some of its meaning to him. These
factors led me to incorporate songs ranging from "The Itsy Bitsy
Spider" to "Go Down, Moses" into our daily work from then on.

VOCABULARY AND THE OLDER CHILD

It had been a long, hard road to reading for eleven-year-old
Cathy, whose mild to moderate hearing loss was compounded
by learning disabilities. Cathy and I celebrated Valentine's Day
by reading her first newspaper article together. It was the story
of a couple whose romance had been kindled by a chance meeting through the fence of a concentration camp. The article
caught my eye because Cathy's class had been reading a novel
about a young girl during the time of the Holocaust. This gave
Cathy the background she needed to make her way through the
article, with some help from me.

This help took the form of vocabulary work that moved
from familiar to unfamiliar concepts. Cathy's level of language
and general knowledge had reached the point that she understood and remembered the verbal explanations that accompanied the making of each card.

Roma used to feed
Herman when they
were children

and she resumed
14 years later.

Herman's parents were killed.

They were <u>exterminated</u>

Herman's life was <u>spared</u>.

Nazi times.

the Nazi <u>era</u>

the Holocaust

---

the Statue of Liberty

Herman's concentration camp was <u>liberated</u>.

---

an <u>epic</u> poem

an <u>epic</u> tale

> " I remember being
> in a walker," recalled
> Cathy.

> Opposites:
>
> ordinary
> extraordinary

KEEPING TRACK

Gillingham and Stillman (1965) state: "It is a great comfort to the pupil for whom all language study has been vague and uncertain, to feel that he is following a precise course of study of which all parts are logically integrated" (p. 120).

Vocabulary development lends itself easily to the regularity of routines. At the children's request, I usually begin each session by going over current vocabulary. Children read their words, illustrating meaning or usage as needed. Missed words are set aside to be reinforced. As they read, children give each word a check in the corner. Words with three checks are considered learned.

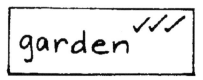

In order to provide variety for children who have been using vocabulary cards year after year, I have introduced different systems for dispensing with words no longer in use. Children have taken their words home, taped them to the refrigerator, or played with them. We have also filed vocabulary cards in a shoebox or index card box in alphabetical order, or by month, with oaktag dividers:

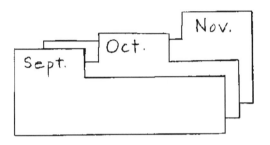

Each method of disposing of "retired" word cards has its advantages. Several children have regularly used old vocabulary cards to play "school" with younger brothers and sisters. Filing words in alphabetical order gives practice in this skill. Filing words by month clearly allows children to see their cumulative vocabulary growth. Interestingly, even minor alterations such as these have been sufficient to sustain children's enthusiasm for vocabulary work from one year to another.

The "Hundred-Square"

An extension of the concept of keeping track has been to duplicate hundred-squares (see example below) and hang up one for each child. Children from first or second grade on enjoy this way of keeping track of the number of words they have mastered. Every day, children count up their words with three checks and color in that number of spaces.

The hundred-square creates an additional possibility for active participation. It also provides tangible evidence of vocabulary growth. As each hundred-square fills up, a new one is taped over it. This offers the opportunity for incidental learning in counting by hundreds, tens, and ones.

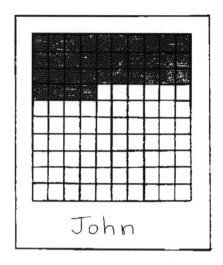

ADDITIONAL SOURCES OF WORD LEARNING

Casual conversation is a rich source of vocabulary and idioms. When Douglas came in sporting a new outfit, we wrote that he was "dressed in blue *from head to toe.*" The same day, he reminisced about a former teacher who had left our school to work closer to home. We jotted down that Ms. H. had had "such a long trip to school" that it just "wasn't *convenient* for her."

Emily, whose favorite color was purple, was scrutinizing several crayons before making her selection. Entitling a card "Different *shades* of purple," we listed lavender, violet, and purple with a patch of color next to each. One day Emily came to the resource room with a case of hiccups. A few minutes later, I got the hiccups myself. From her own experience, Emily was aware that chicken pox were contagious. We took that concept a step further on a card that read: "Chicken pox is *contagious.* Hiccups must be contagious, too!"

It was Emily whose language impairment had all but prevented her from understanding and appreciating *The Courage of Sarah Noble.* This made it especially enjoyable that now, two years later, we were able to use words to explain and enhance a humorous situation in this playful way.

Reading for Concepts (Liddle 1977), the Barnell-Loft *Specific Skills* series (Boning 1976), and other comprehension practice books that are predominantly nonfiction yield important words and concepts related to history and science. Highlighting such words even for a moment on three consecutive days opens up opportunities beyond word recognition.

For example, a teacher can relate a known word to a new context, or associate a new word with a concept already familiar to the child. A word can serve to trigger a child's memory for related words or events. It can be used to generate a list of words or concepts around a common theme. As teachers put into words such cognitive processes as generalizing, inferring, and making associations, they are demonstrating different patterns of abstract thinking. Along with the words themselves, these patterns will take root and become internalized according to the level and ability of the child.

All reading and/or conversation is fertile ground for vocabulary and language development. Words that arise in these situations have a dual advantage. They have their roots in a context that has been illuminated and made meaningful. Equally important, they have grown out of a warm personal interaction between teacher and child.

A Stable Element

Activities come and go, having served their purpose. But vocabulary cards stand out; I have returned to this system year after year with little modification. What sets vocabulary cards apart from other activities in this regard?

The distinguishing feature seems to be the simple, predictable format that allows the process to be used in conjunction with other learning experiences without overshadowing the experiences themselves. As a result, the content of the cards becomes an individual expression of each child's history in any given year.

Duplicating with one child what has worked with another does not often succeed without adaptation. Yet the flexibility inherent in vocabulary cards as a means of expanding word knowledge has allowed this approach to become a stable element of the resource room curriculum.

SUMMARY

A minimal level of input generally suffices for basic language development (Horowitz 1995). Horowitz refers to input beyond the minimum—for example, exposure to rich vocabulary—as "normal extra targeting of environmental input" (p. 13). "Extraordinary targeting of environmental input" is still more focused and more intense. Horowitz notes that "for the child without normal hearing, extraordinary targeting of environmental input will be *required* in order for normal language to develop."

The routines and experiences of daily living offer unparalleled opportunities for language development. The resource room setting is more limited in this regard. Yet the resource room, with its "extraordinary targeting of environmental input," can stimulate language development in all children, some of whom go on to increase their vocabularies through incidental learning.

Chapter 12

Creating a Community of Learners

> *Susie read to Diana and Emily a draft about a chickadee*
> *which came and stood on her outstretched hand, picking*
> *at some seed which she held out for him.*
>
> Amy: *Good! What happens next?*
> Susie: *He looks at me, then quickly hops on my hand.*
> Diane: *How did it feel?*
> Susie: *It tickled . . . not like needles, just a nice, little*
>   *hold.*
> Diane: *I've had that feeling before.*
> Susie: *I didn't realize, but I should add that in.*
> Diane: *I think it adds a lot to your story to tell that.*
> Amy: *Do you need any other help?*
> Susie: *Do you like the lead, or do you think I should*
>   *start it when the chickadee lands on my hand?*
>
> *Calkins (1983, 122)*

This exchange, which took place among three fourth graders, was overheard and recorded by Lucy Calkins during a writing workshop. Because the Columbia University Teachers College Writing Project integrates reading, writing, and language, it stands as one model of a language experience program at work. Peer interaction is a vital part of this process. Children-as-authors conceive their ideas and carry them through in classroom workshops humming with the sounds of writers in all stages of productivity. Children derive inspiration from one another, and learn to consult with each other regarding various aspects of their writing. Similar conditions prevail with regard to the reading and sharing of literature.

DEVELOPING A SENSE OF COMMUNITY
IN THE RESOURCE ROOM

The resource room, in comparison, is often home to only one or two children at a time. They are likely to be impoverished as language users and, consequently, as readers. The individual or small-group sessions are not a luxury, but a necessity, if children are to have a chance of approaching their age and grade levels.

But a one-to-one relationship between teacher and child is very different from a classroom filled with children in close contact with one another and with each other's work. Some aspects of this are impossible to duplicate. Yet I felt that it was important to create, somehow, a community of learners in spite of the fact that most children never actually work together. The following activities have helped bring this goal closer to reality.

Sign-Out Book

Two grants from the Fund for New York City Public Education enabled me to develop a resource room library. As books began to trickle into the resource room, I realized it would be necessary to keep track of them in some way. I wanted the children to borrow them freely, but I didn't want them lost or mislaid. The solution was a sign-out book using a three-ring binder and a duplicated form:

Name	Book	
James	Curious George and the DINOSAUR	✓
Jonathan	BABY BEARS	✓
Melissa	Beanstalk Jack and The	✓
Thomas	Berenstain Bears Go to School	✓
Celina	Go dog go	✓
Jonathan	Little Red Riding hood	✓
Melissa	Pigs	✓
Thomas	Max Found Towsticks	✓
James	sleeping Beauty	✓
Celina	Are you my mommy	✓
Jonathan	STORies Read with me	✓

Children recorded books they borrowed, and checked them off when they brought them back. There was no limit to how long children could keep books, as long as they were still reading or rereading and enjoying them. The sign-out book allowed me to look back and check with children about books that might have been overlooked or forgotten.

The sign-out book served its purpose. An occasional book has been lost and paid for. Very few books have disappeared without a trace.

As time went on, the sign-out book took on an importance beyond its record-keeping function. Children were impressed as page after page filled up with names and titles. This spurred them on in their reading efforts.

Reading continuously and in quantity was a new experience for children who had barely read independently before. As the volume and variety of reading increased, children began to take note of which books their fellow readers were checking out. They were delighted to discover that someone else was reading a book they had previously read and enjoyed. One child would ask another about an unfamiliar title and lay claim to that book when the current reader was finished. In this way, the sign-out book played an unanticipated role in uniting individual readers into a reading community.

Reading Logs

As borrowing and returning books became a way of life, I wanted to make the children's work in reading visible. One day I lined an oversized sheet of paper and wrote "Reading Log" across the top. From then on, the children listed their names with the titles of the books they read.

Children were required to relate their stories to me before adding them to the log. This gave me the chance to evaluate their comprehension and fill in gaps through questioning and discussion. I tried to hear the retelling of stories as we came up the stairs or were putting on FM equipment, the school hearing aids that include teacher-worn microphones (see p. 20). To the extent that I could fit it in, this freed up the resource room sessions for other purposes.

The logs filled up steadily, and by the end of the year, eight or nine of them were lined up across the front of the room.

Thanks to the children's uninhibited use of markers, they were cheerful and eye-catching. As children came into the resource room, they usually went right over to check on the latest entries. Because the logs were collective rather than individual, they were motivating without inviting comparison and competitiveness in a negative sense.

Like the sign-out book, reading logs provided tangible evidence of the children's growth in reading. They welded the children into a group and kept enthusiasm for reading high.

Authors Club

Reading together in the resource room gave children the foundation they needed to begin to read on their own. Their reading, coupled with practice in relating what they had read, produced results in several areas. The children improved in their ability to follow and retain a story line, and to communicate the essence of a story and their responses to it.

In time, the children's acquaintance with literature broadened to the point that each one had read a number of books by specific authors. This led to the formation of the Authors Club. Children who read three or more books by a given author listed reader, author, and titles on an Authors Club form which they added to the bulletin board.

Filling out a form and stapling it up on the board were the sole requirements for membership in the "club." It was satisfying to see the board fill up with these sheets, which attested to the children's budding awareness of authors and their works.

A new level of thinking about literature was now within reach. Different authors wrote books that differed in length and format. Some authors leaned toward particular settings. The Authors Club brought to children's awareness different threads that connected story to story, author to author. Many conversations about reading and writing began with "This reminds me of. . . ."

The Authors Club bulletin board supplemented the Reading Log wall as a center of interest. Children's acquaintance with a particular author was reinforced and extended when they saw familiar and not-yet familiar titles on another child's list. It was always exciting to discover that someone else was "into" a favorite author. The display provided a basis for helping children branch out in their reading: "If you enjoyed *Pippi Longstocking,* you might really love. . . ."

```
Authors   Club

Reader:_____

Author:_____

Books
  1. _____
  2. _____
  3. _____
```

Illustrators Club

Curtis was an artistically talented boy with a special sensitivity to beauty. He was very taken by Susan Jeffer's illustrations of *Hansel and Gretel* (Grimm 1980). His face lit up when I handed him another fairy tale she had illustrated. This gave me the idea of adding an Illustrators Club section to our bulletin board.

The Illustrators Club boosted enthusiasm for reading. It gave us another forum for expanding language and using it to compare, contrast, and make associations. Like the Authors Club, it stimulated reading and deepened the bonds among readers.

```
Illustrators   Club

Reader:_____

Illustrator:
         _____

Books
  1. _____
  2. _____
```

Theme Club

I don't remember exactly what sparked the birth of the third and last of our clubs. It was some moment of recognition—mine or a child's—that two different books had something important in common. The Theme Club gave us a way of looking at literature with new eyes. Plots, settings, and character traits were all food for thought.

I had never expected to reach the point of our being able to reflect on reading in this way. When the time came, the difficulties turned out to be in my own mind. The children found it surprisingly easy to follow along and answer such questions as, "Can you think of any other story about a person who makes a sacrifice to help someone else? What other character do you know who is into solving mysteries? What do Sarah Noble and Laura Ingalls Wilder have in common?"

```
Theme Club

Reader: _____

Books:
   1. _____
   2. _____

Theme: _____
_____
_____
_____
_____ _____
```

Throughout the year, I continued to ask leading questions in order to bring different and more subtle kinds of associations to light. Some of the children began to perceive threads among stories on their own.

The children had advanced from being severely limited in their reading ability to becoming conversant about authors, illustrators, and themes. This was an exciting and rewarding group landmark.

SELECTING BOOKS

As the children progressed in reading, they seldom left the resource room without making sure they had a book for the evening and several for the weekend. Interestingly, they did not avoid books that challenged them. Even Shelley, who tended to stay well within her comfort level, slowly found her way to chapter books she could read and enjoy.

Some children made their selections by taking home the first books that came into their hands, regardless of level or content. As a result, they frequently returned books unread. I learned to explain that the way to tell whether a book was right for them was to sit down with it, open to the first page, and read quietly for a few minutes. This approach gives children a basis for deciding whether to persevere with a book or put it back. It also seems less judgmental than informing children a book is too hard, enabling them to make the decision for themselves. Further, it leaves room for the possibility that a book which does not match their interests or reading levels at the present time might turn out to be just the book for them at another time.

Still, children occasionally returned books that were too hard or "not right" for them. Sometimes the stumbling block was a matter of style. A few sessions of collaborative reading accustomed their ears to longer and more complex sentences or to a subtle humor that had eluded them, and enabled them to move forward on their own.

PICTURE BOOKS

At the same time, the children continued to read quantities of picture books. Their delight in picture books, both easy and more sophisticated, reflected their growing competence in reading. It also seemed to meet a need to intersperse reading that required effort with more relaxing interludes. The intensity of the children's attraction to picture books conveyed the feeling that perhaps they were making up for those early years, when they had lacked the language and reading competence to enjoy the stories that are part of many young children's lives.

Picture books came to the fore once again with the introduction of higher level thinking skills. Listing the collected works of H. A. Rey on an Authors Club form gave *Curious George* new status. Becoming acquainted with illustrators drew attention to the works of Maurice Sendak, Garth Williams, and others.

Picture books were rich in the same themes that run through all great literature. Friendship is celebrated in *Frog and Toad* (Lobel 1995) and *Amigo* (Baylor 1989). Patience and determination triumph in *The Carrot Seed* (Krauss 1989) and in *A Chair for My Mother* (Williams 1982). Children gain acceptance in *Crow Boy* (Yashima 1976) and in *William's Doll* (Zolotow 1985).

Examining picture books from these points of view invested them with fresh interest. It gave children the means to step back and read in an active and perhaps less naive way than do very young children. This brought picture books into an age-appropriate context for these older elementary school children.

The resource room setting does not always lend itself to communal involvement. Sometimes, however, resource room life can be structured so as to put children in touch with one another as readers and writers. This leads to results that would not have been possible had each child been engaged in solitary pursuits.

Chapter 13

Poetry

Poetry anthologies, from Mother Goose to collections by particular poets, were part of our resource room library. I have found that the sounds, cadence, rhyme, and whimsical language that delight small children are not easily absorbed or appreciated by most young deaf and hard-of-hearing children. In addition, the many demands on resource room time have taken precedence over developing an appreciation of poetry as children become older.

THE POETRY BOX

Realizing this, I ended up introducing poetry in an unexpected way. It happened as the result of browsing through several collections of poems for children in a small-town library. These old anthologies contained a wide variety of poetry, including epic poems several pages long. I duplicated several dozen poems representing a range of forms, content, and feelings. I mounted them on halfsheets of colored card stock and put them in a "Poetry Box."

I made the Poetry Box available to three sixth graders. The children's vocabularies and use of language were at least adequate. One of the children was Crystal, with her rich idiomatic language. Another was Curtis, the "King of Tornadoes," whose head had felt like "the solar system going around."

The children were fairly well acquainted with children's literature, and had been exposed to a range of styles and content. Each child had had experience expressing his or her own thoughts in writing, and had experimented with a variety of writing styles. I felt guardedly optimistic that this background would provide the foundation these twelve-year-olds needed to enjoy and appreciate poetry.

Incorporating poetry at this stage was feasible from the point of view of resource room programming. Because the children's language level was relatively solid, I no longer felt it necessary to be cautious about introducing activities that would take away from time needed for developing basic language. Poetry could now be worked in as part of the children's ongoing language development, with time left over for academic support.

From time to time, the children would leaf through the cards and choose poems that captured their interests. We read and enjoyed numerous poems together. Some were memorized. The following poems were among the children's favorites.

CITY
In the morning the city
Spreads its wings
Making a song
In stone that sings.

In the evening the city
Goes to bed
Hanging lights
About its head.
    Langston Hughes

WHO HAS SEEN THE WIND
Who has seen the wind?
Neither I nor you;
But when the leaves hang
    trembling
The wind is passing through.

Who has seen the wind?
Neither you nor I;
But when the trees bow down
    their heads
The wind is passing by.
    Christina Rossetti

THIS IS THE KEY
This is the key of the kingdom:
In that kingdom there is a city.
In that city there is a town.
In that town there is a street.
In that street there is a lane.
In that lane there is a yard.
In that yard there is a house.
In that house there is a room.
In that room there is a bed.
On that bed there is a basket.
In that basket there are some
    flowers.
Flowers in a basket.

THE PRAYER OF THE OLD HORSE
See, Lord,
my coat hangs in tatters,
like homespun, old, threadbare.
All that I had of zest,
all my strength,
I have given in hard work
and kept nothing back for myself.
Now
my poor head swings
to offer up all the loneliness of my
    heart.
Dear God,
stiff on my thickened legs

Basket on the bed.
Bed in the room.
Room in the house.
House in the yard.
Yard in the lane.
Lane in the street.
Street in the town.
Town in the city.
City in the kingdom.
Of the kingdom this is the key.
          Anonymous

I stand here before You:
Your unprofitable servant.
Oh! Of Your goodness,
give me a gentle death.
Amen.
          Carmen Bernos de Gasztold

The fact that poetry was approached in an incidental way had advantages and disadvantages. The children developed only a nodding acquaintance with a handful of poets and their work. At the same time, it was a stimulating and pleasurable experience, and closer than we had ever come before to having a taste of different kinds of poetry.

CROSSING THE THRESHOLD

In describing his experience teaching delinquent boys, Fader (1976) writes that "semiliterate readers do not need semiliterate books . . . 'Reading' is a peculiarly personal interaction between a reader and a book . . . But *in no case* does this interaction demand an understanding of every word by the reader. In fact, the threshold of understanding—of meaningful interaction—is surprisingly low, and even in many complex books can be pleasurably crossed by many simple readers" (pp. 95–96).

At no time was this truth more apparent than in the children's reading of poetry. The most interesting surprise for me was twelve-year-old Curtis' preference for the long epic and narrative poems, which I had hesitated to include at all. With the help of a tape of the text, Curtis committed himself to memorizing several lengthy stanzas from Edgar Allan Poe's "The Raven." He then undertook the saga of Robin Hood.

ROBIN HOOD AND THE BISHOP OF HEREFORD
Come, gentlemen all, and listen a while;
   A story to you I'll unfold —-
How Robin Hood served the Bishop,
   When he robb'd him of his gold.

As it befel in merry Barnsdale,
  And under the green-wood tree,
The Bishop of Hereford was to come by,
  With all his companye.

'Come, kill a ven'son,' said bold Robin Hood,
  'Come, kill me a good fat deer;
The Bishop's to dine with me today,
  And he shall pay well for his cheer.

'We'll kill a fat ven'son,' said bold Robin Hood,
  'And dress't by the highway-side,
And narrowly watch for the Bishop,
  Lest some other way he should ride . . .'

The drama and story line were exciting to Curtis, and he loved the numerous readings and rereadings it took for the old poetic language to become comfortably familiar. Learning chunks of those particular poems by heart required concentration and perseverance.

Curtis' success in making the language of poetry his own illustrates a discrepancy that sometimes exists between a child's independent reading level and his or her instructional level—the level at which the child reads with comprehension given the needed support. On a vocabulary-oriented standardized test, Curtis scored only in the sixth percentile. This reflects the influence of his moderate hearing loss, compounded by limited exposure to English outside of school. Yet Curtis' demonstrated ability belies his reading score. Accomplishments such as his allow us to share Vygotsky's conviction that "what a child can do in cooperation today, he can do alone tomorrow" (Vygotsky 1962, 104).

As poems were memorized, children copied them in their best handwriting and put them up on the hall bulletin board. This group display gave children the impetus to select and tackle poem after poem. Slowly the board filled up with poetry. It was a satisfying achievement.

Chapter 14

Facilitating Writing

The road to reading had begun with a variety of activities aimed at developing decoding and comprehension skills. My hope was that these activities would give children the language and fluency they needed to read with ease and enjoyment. As time went on, it became apparent that this was not happening. This lack of movement and direction prompted me to look further, and led to the "my turn, your turn" experiment in reading.

A similar situation prevailed with regard to writing. In the earliest grades, children had begun to write using a combination of sight words and phonics knowledge. By third grade, they were doing fairly well on spelling tests, but were barely able to write simple sentences.

THE YOUNG DEAF OR HARD-OF-HEARING WRITER

Young children are generally well grounded in language by the time they begin learning to write. Children who have acquired basic vocabulary and sentence structure have the language they need to express their thoughts in writing. It is this grounding in language that enabled Ashton-Warner's five-year-old pupils to move from single words to two or three sentences of autobiographical writing: "I went to the river and I kissed Lily and I ran away. Then I kissed Phillipa. Then I ran away and went for a swim" (Ashton-Warner 1963, 53).

The Maori children of Ashton-Warner's day, with their cultural and language differences, needed a bridge from the known to the unknown. Working from the "inner man outward" (p. 62), Ashton-Warner created a basis that would carry them forward into all kinds of reading. Reading and writing took on cultural relevance when drawn from children's own stories about family and village life. Thoughts flowed freely as children gained knowledge of the mechanics of writing. Six-year-olds wrote half a page, seven-year-olds a page or more a day.

Several factors are likely to interfere with the flow of written language when the young writer is deaf or hard of hearing:

- The number and variety of words available for writing is limited by the child's sight vocabulary.
- Hearing-impaired children perceive, and therefore articulate, many sounds in an incomplete and/or distorted way. This gives them fewer reliable clues when they begin to write. While discrimination and articulation can be developed with auditory training and speech therapy, this takes time.
- Many deaf and hard-of-hearing children who have not had the benefit of early language development are introduced to writing at a time when they are just beginning to acquire language. Vocabulary alone does not give children the ability to express themselves in connected language. The delay in moving beyond single words to meaningful connected writing can persist long past the age of Ashton-Warner's young writers and those in countless early childhood classrooms.

Children who enter the resource room with poor verbal skills have been bystanders rather than informed participants in family and other life experiences. A skill as basic as having a conversation may form the core of resource room work for many months (see Chapter 2). Language and experiential deficits are reflected in children's difficulty expressing their thoughts in writing. The development of sight vocabulary, auditory skills, and phonics knowledge helps children master classroom spelling assignments. However, in the absence of a language foundation, none of these leads automatically to personally meaningful writing. As children begin to write, it becomes imperative to find ways of working that will help them gain competence in the mechanics of writing and, ultimately, enable them to use writing to express their thoughts and feelings.

BEGINNING THE PROCESS

Different children require different kinds of help as they struggle to articulate their ideas and express them in writing.

Children often doubt the worth and interest of their own everyday experiences. Again and again it became necessary to engage children in conversation, wait for a sentence that makes their eyes light up, and prod them to "take that sentence out of your mouth and put it on the paper."

A number of strategies proved useful in overcoming specific problems. In every instance, the teacher's guidance gave shape and structure to the learning situation. Some learning opportunities grew out of conversational exchanges based on reading or on topics of interest. This kind of spontaneous yet teacher-directed learning characterizes a whole language approach. Other activities were created and initiated by the teacher in response to specific needs. Meeting these needs gave children skills that would carry over into more natural language learning situations.

A variety of activities that have moved children closer to meaningful writing are illustrated in the following vignettes.

Tape Recorder to the Rescue

Hearing aids coupled with auditory training bring the use of the tape recorder into the realm of the possible for many deaf and hard-of-hearing children. Seven-year-old Belinda had difficulty finding anything at all to talk about. Jerry, her classmate and resource room partner, was an uncommunicative little boy who responded in monosyllables and never initiated a spontaneous exchange. Generating a flow of personal stories was a necessary prerequisite to writing for these two second graders. The tape recorder suggested itself as a possibility because both children were capable of expressing themselves in connected language.

The fascination of dictating into a tape recorder freed these children as I had not been able to do. After a month of reciting their stories into a microphone and listening to themselves on tape, Belinda and Jerry began to greet me with happenings from home and to relate parts of books they had read. This verbal communication became a basis for writing.

Building Language and Memory: Auditory-Kinesthetic Reinforcement

As a second grader with a history of significant language impairment, Emily would sometimes volunteer one-sentence news tidbits ("I went to the park"), but could not elaborate on them. Emily's difficulty was twofold. Even with guidance it was not easy for her to expand on her own stories. In addition, she was unable to remember even a two-sentence sequence.

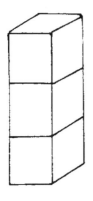

Natural language activities had not succeeded in strengthening Emily's memory, or in helping her to relate experiences in greater detail. It seemed possible that supplementing whole language activities with a structured, multisensory approach could offer Emily the help she needed.

We began by using inch-cubes, one for each sentence, to build a tower. At first it was necessary to ask leading questions to elicit each sentence. Before too long, Emily was able to build three- and four-sentence block towers with a minimum of prompting.

Once the tower was built, Emily touched each block and recalled the sentence it represented. This was challenging, and it took weeks of practice before she was able to use her memory to reconstruct her story.

At this point, we moved from inch-cubes to 3″ x 5″ rectangles of colored felt. This technique (Bell 1986) provides a kinesthetic aid to memory. As part of a sequence of activities designed to develop language comprehension and thinking ability, the teacher elicits a verbal description of a simple illustration. Each time the child is about to formulate a sentence, the teacher lays another piece of felt on the table. As the child speaks, he or she touches the felt rectangle. The child then retells the five- or six-sentence story, touching the felt pieces in sequence. In my work with Emily, I excerpted and adapted this aspect of Bell's visualizing-verbalizing technique.

My goal in the resource room was to enable Emily to formulate and write a three-sentence experience story independently. She would articulate one sentence, touching the first rectangle. Then another sentence, touching the second rectangle. Then back to the beginning, touching each rectangle and saying the two sentences in order. Then the third rectangle, the third sentence, and back to the beginning for a cumulative run-through. Now she was ready to write.

At the beginning, Emily needed me to refresh her memory frequently. As the weeks went on, her concentration and memory became stronger. After about two months of this work, there began to be a noticeable improvement in her language-writing ability. She could almost toss off reciting a three-sentence sequence, and writing was no longer such a burden for her. I began leaving the table to encourage her to carry through on her own. Spelling aside, she began writing more fluently, with few alterations or omissions.

The situation was different in the more distracting classroom environment. While most of the children were writing a page or more, Emily was likely to be staring into space with half a sentence on her paper. This persisted until, one day, she produced a page-long story about a ghost-man who lived "deep, deep in the forest." It was the first sign that Emily's new-found abilities to focus and retain were transferring to situations in which they were needed.

A combination of factors contributed to this success: an experienced classroom teacher; resource room support; a mother who had come to acknowledge and accept her daughter's difficulties and had begun to take a more active part in the child's language development; and Emily's recent affiliation with an experienced learning disabilities tutor.

Awakening Memory

Along with her difficulty finding topics of interest, Belinda was unable to hold a sentence in her memory long enough to finish writing it. Shelley, a fourth grader, had a similar problem. She could rattle off a list of after-school activities, which evaporated as soon as she picked up her pencil to write about them. Both of these children were helped by dictating stories into the tape recorder, then using the "rewind" button to check back and refresh their memories as often as necessary. As time went on, they gradually became able to get started on their own and to write several sentences without prompting.

Emily's difficulties had been so severe that they did not respond to a whole language approach without supplementary activities of a highly structured, multisensory nature. Belinda and Shelley were helped by the simpler intervention of the tape recorder. If this had not worked, it would have been necessary to explore further.

THE DRAWING PATH TO WRITING

In contrast to the children described above, eight-year-old Cynthia had an unimpaired memory and expressed herself in fluent, though ungrammatical English. Her difficulty was in the area of writing itself.

One morning, Cynthia came in very upset about having missed the bus the day before. She related a whole series of events, from looking out the window and running downstairs to watching the bus disappear around the corner. While her language was adequate, her writing skills were nearly nonexistent.

I expected that Cynthia's rich inner language would enable her to draw detailed pictures based on this experience. Drawing four-picture sequence stories helped ease this severely hard-of-hearing girl into writing. With her story organized and laid out before her, she participated in captioning each picture—first orally, then in writing. This approach reduced writing to a manageable format and made it possible to begin work on basic writing skills.

CONVERSATIONS IN WRITING

"You know how we have conversations back and forth—first my turn to talk, then your turn? We're going to have a conversation with our pencils. I'll start."

Children who are reluctant to write because writing is such a chore for them have responded with pleasure to written dialogues. At age ten, Robert had the skills needed to express himself in writing. On his own, however, he seldom persevered past two or three sentences.

How are you doing today?
fine and how are you doing today?
Well, the battery in my
watch died at 7:10 this
morning and I was almost
late for school / wow yesterday
I had had to take the train to
school because the bus did not
pick me up. And I had to walk
from 9th ave and 16th. No
kidding / Who brought you?
Nobody I came by myself. I'm

> impressed. Was this your _____
> first time taking public
> transportation on your own?
> NO because one time I came
> from my grandma house by
> my self and that was my
> first. You're getting to be
> so independent. Do you feel
> ready for a train pass? Well
> I can't because pat said I
> have to can sell the school bus
> and my mothe said no. Maybe
> when you're in junior high...

Folktales and fairytales have provided a basis for collaborative writing. Dialogue and narrative combined in this retelling of *Hansel and Gretel*. A second-grade girl with a limited command of English alternated between writing her own sentences and dictating sentences for me to write:

> Stepmother: lets take The
> children far far away and
> leave Them There.
>
> Gretel: I'm scared, Hansel.
>
> Hansel: don't be scared, I
> will take care of you,
>
> Hansel picked up the
> pebbles. He put Them in His
> pocket. The step Mother and
> The father took The children
> in to The woods. Hansel
> dropped the pebbles.
> Hansel and Gretel followed The
> pebbles all The way home.

Written conversations have the same benefits as collaborative reading. They move writing along at a relatively rapid pace with children who find writing difficult. They reduce the tediousness inherent in writing at this stage, since children have to struggle with only a sentence or two before relaxing while I respond to what they have written.

In the dialogue situation, writing becomes a satisfying means of communication, in which spelling and sentence structure are subordinate but essential elements. For a description of incorporating teacher direction in the writing process, see Chapter 15 "Behind the Scenes."

Several factors contribute to the success of this approach to writing.

- Children write about what they know.
- The process of alternating sentences keeps the momentum going.
- Children can count on the teacher to prevent a difficult task from becoming burdensome.
- Teacher and child are equal partners in an undertaking of mutual interest.

The skill, confidence, and pleasure gained from written conversations have helped bring children closer to independent writing.

A "BACKWARDS" APPROACH

Tom had entered third grade with a severe hearing loss and lack of exposure to English outside of school. In spite of Tom's enthusiasm and sense of purpose, his language was very slow in developing. His love of learning and interest in history and science were far ahead of his language and reading skills. Writing was the most difficult of all areas, and the most frustrating. He hated to write.

What helped was a kind of "backwards" approach to writing. We would begin with a discussion of some aspect of our collaborative reading. I listened for a portion of conversation that formed a short but cohesive unit. I formulated a question to fit this information. I told Tom that I was going to write a question in his notebook, and that he would answer with what he had just told me.

Even this was tough going because of Tom's difficulty with English and with the mechanics of writing. Personal narratives might have been less demanding at this point. I persevered with writing related to science and history because of Tom's clear and intense interest in both areas. These writing experiences honored his seriousness of purpose as a learner, while giving him a glimpse of what he might be able to do one day more independently.

> What did James Watt
> and Marconi have
> in common when
> they were young?
>
> James Watt when he was
> small he wanted to learn
> more about Steam. When
> Marconi was little, he wanted
> to learne more about electricy
>
> Describe Marconi's ex-
> periment with the bell.
>
> He attached the wire to th top
> of the house and he attached the
> other end to the bell. The lightning
> hit the wire and made the bell
> ring. Marconi excited because his
> expeliment worked. He was disappointed
> because no one in his family was
> care about it.

STRUCTURE AND/OR NATURAL? A SYNTHESIS

Like most resource room activities, this apparently spontaneous approach to writing contained elements that were deliberately and carefully structured.

- The text had been selected by me, based on my knowledge of Tom's passionate interest in science. It was my judgment that the biography, which was well above his independent reading level, would be within Tom's grasp as we read and discussed together. I reasoned that the somewhat laborious pace the book would require would be offset by Tom's interest in Marconi's boyhood love of science and his accomplishments throughout his life.
- The discussion that accompanied our reading grew partly out of Tom's own questions and reactions, and partly out

of my attempts to expand his language and understanding. Tom's written answers were basically his own. Yet from time to time I offered him the language he needed or provided a listening exercise to help him discriminate the sounds needed for correct spelling. At times my input served as a reminder of what Tom already knew but had only partially consolidated. At other times, I took advantage of opportunities to introduce new information and language concepts.

This teaching-learning experience was engendered by Tom's interest and sustained by his enthusiasm. I made the reading accessible to him by clarifying unfamiliar language and concepts and by linking Tom's previous knowledge with information in Marconi's biography. The structure inherent in every aspect of the activity was tailored to Tom's learning needs in two ways. First, it provided a scaffold for the development of vocabulary, grammar, syntax, and auditory skills. Second, it allowed me to elicit Tom's own language and reduce it to a quantity and format Tom could record in writing without feeling intolerably frustrated or overwhelmed.

In working with children with remedial needs, I have become less inclined to conceive of structure and natural language as opposing, or even complementary, approaches. In Tom's "backwards" approach to writing, as in virtually all resource room activities, the distinction blurs. Spontaneity and structure merge into a way of teaching that responds to children's multifaceted needs, while stimulating further learning. Writing, perhaps the most difficult of all undertakings for language-delayed deaf and hard-of-hearing children, has been well served by this synthesis.

SYLLABLE BY SYLLABLE

In order to incorporate phonics information into their reading and writing, children need to be able to:

- distinguish one syllable from another;
- discern the sequence of sounds in each syllable; and
- recognize and supply the letter or combination of letters that represent each sound.

The rules of syllable division based on the Orton Gillingham approach (see Chapter 18) have provided a basis for our work in this area. The following example illustrates the first of three syllable division patterns.

- Identify the vowels with a dot above each.   m å g nė t

- Connect the dots.   m $\overline{\text{å g}}$ nė t

- Label the vowels, and the consonants between them.   v c c v
  m $\overline{\text{å g}}$ nė t

- Draw a vertical line between the two consonants.   v c | c v
  m å g | nė t

This reduces the word to a series of short, manageable units.

Syllable Division and Writing

Writing poses an additional problem. Children need to learn to separate words into syllables before attempting to write words they do not know how to spell. This is a realistic goal for some deaf and most hard-of-hearing children. Using inch-cubes as a visual aid has enabled children to hear and spell sounds and syllables accurately.

To introduce this activity, I put a handful of wooden inch-sized cubes on the table. I choose a word that has come up while working or in conversation:

"In the word 'dentist,' how many syllables?" I exaggerate the spaces between syllables, putting up first one, then two fingers as I pronounce each syllable.

I repeat the word, sliding one inch-cube in front of the child for each syllable. We chant "den-tist" as I point to each block.

I point to the blocks in order. The children enunciate one syllable at a time. I point to the blocks at random. "What's the first syllable of 'dentist'? The second syllable?"

This introduction serves as preparation for writing.

"Now we're going to write 'dentist.' What's the first sylla-ble of 'den-tist'? How do you spell / den /?" The child spells the syllable orally, then writes it.

"What's the second syllable? How do you spell / tist /?"

As the process becomes established, we practice four or five words daily or every other day. Less frequent formal prac-tice remains an ongoing part of resource room sessions as chil-dren add new letter combinations to their spelling repertoire.

"How Do You Spell . . .?"

What begins as drill joins other strategies that are called on as needed. When a child asks for help in spelling a word, we take out the inch-cubes. Sometimes with help and sometimes independently, children use this aid to hearing and articulating sounds more clearly. Spelling often follows easily.

When words contain sounds that children have not yet learned to spell, two responses are possible. For a child with a firm knowledge of the spelling he or she has learned so far, this may be a natural opportunity to introduce the new sound and its spelling. In contrast, I tend simply to give the spelling of a word or syllable to a child who is still in the process of integrating previously learned letter-sound correspondences.

A variation that children love is to practice syllable division in their notebooks using drawings rather than actual blocks. Using the process described above, children write each syllable under the appropriate block. Children who are relatively advanced in their vocabularies and knowledge of spelling love the challenge of four- and even five-syllable words.

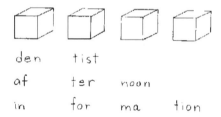

den   tist

af   ter   noon

in   for   ma   tion

Drawing each block with a different colored pencil and having children write each syllable in that color renews children's enthusiasm for a task that demands concentration and repetition.

SOMETHING BORROWED . . .

Hearing and sequencing the sounds within syllables require fine auditory discrimination. A simple strategy has helped children focus on sounds and sound clusters that are difficult for them to hear. This way of working is adapted from the Glass Analysis method of teaching children to read words of increasing length (Glass Analysis material is available from Easier to Learn, Adelphi University, Garden City, NJ 11530). The strategy consists of a pair of related questions:

• In the word *bat*, what letter makes the sound of /b/?

- In the word *bat*, what sound does the *b* make?

This questioning can be applied to diphthongs and digraphs, and has been effective in helping children hear consonant blends:

- In the word *town*, what two letters make the sound of /ou/?
- In the word *town*, what sound does *ow* make?

This approach can also be applied to a troublesome syllable within a multisyllabic word such as *farther*: "In the syllable /ther/, what two letters make the sound of /er/?"

Some sounds are likely to be difficult to hear for most children with hearing impairments. The clarity of other sounds varies from child to child depending on his or her audiogram (see Chapter 3). Focusing on a difficult sound in this way for several sessions has improved children's ability to discriminate that sound individually and in a sound sequence.

SOMETHING OLD, SOMETHING NEW

Vocabulary cards, Bell's Visualizing-Verbalizing strategy, Glass Analysis, and the Orton Gillingham approach to teaching phonics are among the techniques of other educators that have become part of resource room practice. Each has contributed an important piece or body of knowledge to my teaching experience. Taking every opportunity to become acquainted with other teachers' ways of working has increased the number of activities and ideas available for use as the need arises.

Some teaching techniques are enhanced by the use of teacher-made or thoughtfully selected commercial material. At the same time, an excess of teaching materials leaves little scope for the child's own imagination and resources. In my experiences, the most valuable materials have been those made with children in conjunction with particular learning needs.

In this spirit, I rarely save teaching material from one year to another. Rather than relying on activities that have worked in the past, my preference has been to make a fresh start in every learning situation. Considering children's needs without preconceived solutions allows for a variety of possibilities.

- *Learning a new approach.* Cathy's reading disability, which had not responded to my best efforts, was finally reversed with the help of the Orton Gillingham approach (see Chapter 18).

- *Inventing a new strategy.* The "Backwards Approach" (see p. 124) that encouraged Tom to persist in expressing his thoughts in writing did not resemble anything I had ever tried before.

- *Duplicating a successful activity.* A way of working that has been effective with another child may fit the current situation better than any other solution. In this case, there is no reason not to use it. Selecting a previously used activity, when it fits a child's needs, is different from re-using an approach without being open to other possibilities. Using inch-cubes to help children hear and spell syllables (see pp. 127–28) has achieved this goal with numerous children with little need for modification.

- *Blending old and new.* Vocabulary cards were derived from the work of two other educators. Expanding on this approach to develop grammar, syntax, and general knowledge created a blend of "borrowed" and original ideas. Similarly, it is possible to blend two approaches of one's own to meet a child's needs.

Every successful teaching experience becomes part of a teacher's growing stock of techniques and strategies, from which ever-changing possibilities suggest themselves.

Chapter 15

Moving Forward in Writing

Writing Project workshops offer children the opportunity to be affected by the enthusiasm and intensity of their fellow writers. As children become absorbed in subjects of their own choosing, they gather language and information germane to their topics and projects. A well-timed suggestion such as "Write down everything you notice about . . ." helps children free themselves of writer's block. Asking what draws a child to a particular topic at a particular time opens the way to new understanding.

SEARCHING FOR MEANING

In many whole language classrooms, writers' notebooks are at the heart of children's work in writing. They contain thoughts, feelings, and observations in various stages of development.

Sometimes independently, sometimes with guidance, children gain sparks of insight from the interconnection of seemingly unrelated thoughts. As new entries are generated by earlier ones, even young children can be helped to perceive chains of thought that run like threads through their entries. A seven-year-old girl, writing about letting her hamster go in the park, reflected that she had "no-one to come home to." At her teacher's suggestion, she looked through her notebook for other fragments that might be connected with this one. The child uncovered an entry about her grandmother: "Before she died, I had someone." Having made the connection between her hamster and her grandmother, the little girl could begin to gather and explore related images around this topic (Calkins 1991, 74–75).

Group Log

Tape recorders, drawings, and other interventions have helped children move beyond their early inability to express themselves on paper. Yet support is still required in every aspect of writing. An activity is needed that does not demand independence in writing before children are ready. It needs to provide a relaxed and encouraging atmosphere for children who find writing difficult and are inclined to write as little as possible.

The answer at various times has been a collective writing log. Every day, each of us contributes an entry to the log. Mine comes first. Each child adds his or hers as the day goes on.

Making myself part of the log has proven beneficial in two ways. Children pounce on the log to get their daily glimpses into Ms. Stelling's life. They also relish the other children's latest news. More importantly, they begin to understand that writing grows out of the happenings of our everyday lives.

This truth does not take root quickly or easily. It has often been difficult to get past the children's initial response that they have nothing to write about. What has worked best is getting them started on writing before this issue has a chance to come up. Casual conversation often provides ideas that can be set down in writing and elaborated on. We chat as we come up the stairs, through the halls, and into the resource room itself:

"You helped your mother bake cookies?"
"Don't tell me your bus came late *again*!"

I react with enthusiasm, hoping to transmit to the children a sense of the value of their own life experiences.

Support of various kinds is required as children begin to write. Help might be needed in coming up with an idea, expanding a word or phrase into a complete sentence, or pushing beyond one or two sentences to three or four. Children need encouragement to apply their newly acquired knowledge of plurals, verb tenses, and other aspects of language. It might be necessary to supply a crucial word that is missing from a child's vocabulary.

As time goes on, children begin to come to the resource room knowing what they are going to write about. Little by little, they come closer to being able to take on the whole process from start to finish. A spiral notebook served as a group log for this group of second- and third-grade children.

Tuesday

Ms. Stelling: Poor Ms. Giffone!
Yesterday I went to
visit her. She is sick.
She has the flu. She
might not be able to
come to school all week.

Tom: It is chinese New Year. My
Grandmother burns incense. I like the
smell. I burn the money, So much
money! not real money. It is make believe
money.

Crystal: Ms. Giffone is absant To D ny.
There is an Other tecer and j coms.

Shelley: My couss'n name is Rocky.
Rocky and I were selling cookies
outsde. Rocky and I heard yelling
It was my mommy. Then I
waved Then I was runing
To her.

Dominique: I went to the movies last
Saturday with my father and my
sister the man over his lade
in the movie they were crsing in the
movie.

Curtis: A long long time ago we
were go on a trip with Mrs. Epps.
and Dominique and me and the rest of
the Clas We saw a big giant wale on the trip.

Individual Logs

The group log, which went on for a year, was followed by individual logs. Because the children still needed a great deal of encouragement and assistance, much of their writing was done in the resource room.

Every month I compiled their stories into a booklet, using two pieces of stiff blackboard and two large rings.

As the monthly logs accumulated, they were hung on hooks along the blackboard ledge. Children enjoyed borrowing them and reading one another's stories.

New year's Eve I waited and waited til twelve o'dock then I heard a lot of people were playing music it is so loud I saw it is eleven fifty nine one minute more it will be twelve. At twelve o'clock we hug and kissed each other. I think I enjoyed New year's eve.

(Cynthia)

January 11, 1990

Today I am going to walk home all by my self for the first time. What I mean is that the bus driver is going to drop me at the after school program after that I'm supposed to walk home. I'm very glad that I'm going to walk home.

Erystal

Weekly Essays

The following September, I looked for a new format that would encourage children to move toward writing more independently. I gave each child a space on the bulletin board for "weekly essays." Every Friday children tacked their latest essays up on the board on top of their previous work. At the end of the month I took them down, typed and duplicated them, and gave each child a booklet of that month's collected essays.

ERRORS IN WRITING: ADDRESS OR IGNORE?

For deaf and hard-of-hearing children, the systematic development of grammar and syntax is a fundamental need. Deficits in these areas, not always obvious during conversation, become apparent in writing.

With some children, grammatical and syntactical errors that have been overcome in oral language may persist in the early stages of writing. Errors typically occur in the use of regular and irregular plurals (two bird, three mouse); and regular and irregular past (Our parakeet die.) Children commonly omit *s* in the possessive (My friend lunchbox); *s* in the third person singular (My brother like to sing); auxiliary verbs (Nelson crying); and definite and indefinite articles (Mommy bought me new coat).

Opportunities to develop and expand language concepts arise naturally as children write. At the same time, overemphasizing accuracy at the expense of content and spontaneity is a disservice to any young writer.

I have found that a seemingly disproportionate amount of teacher input may be required to launch children into writing at a stage at which both content and mechanics are just beyond the child's reach (see Douglas' "tree story" later in this chapter.) This input helps children acquire the skill and confidence they need to begin writing on their own.

Once children reach the point of attempting their first tentative sentences of personally meaningful writing, direction and structure become less important than the child's own felt needs. These range from having words spelled and sentences rephrased so as to express what the child wants to say, to the moral support that conveys confidence in the child's ability to write as well as approval of the writing itself. It takes a long time for independent writing to attain the content and accuracy of the earlier, teacher-assisted writing. Every writing experience strengthens the child's ability and self-reliance, and moves him or her closer to this level.

As children gain ease and fluency in writing, it becomes important to expand language concepts and to develop and refine grammar, syntax, and punctuation. This point is reached when children are comfortable enough and proficient enough in expressing their thoughts, that their interest and attention can be directed toward editing without compromising the spontaneous flow of language and ideas (see "Learning to Edit" later in this chapter).

EVALUATING GROWTH IN WRITING

One spring, I had the privilege of conferring on a regular basis with a Writing Project consultant assigned to my school. In order to make optimum use of our first session, I had prepared thumbnail sketches of the children as readers and writers. Years later, I came across those reading-writing profiles.

I was amazed. I had long forgotten what the children had been like only a few years before. At that time, I was feeling stymied about twelve-year-old Crystal, who had showed promise as a reader and writer, yet whose genuineness and vitality were conspicuously absent from her current work. Reading her profile reminded me that she had begun to lose initiative years earlier, perhaps in response to a lack of emotional support at home.

In contrast, an eleven-year-old severely hard-of-hearing girl had begun to write fluently and spontaneously. Though Cynthia's language was not yet grammatically or syntactically accurate, my own description brought me back to the days when writing a simple sentence had been beyond her. This put her developing awareness of verb tense and run-on sentences in a more encouraging light.

Reading the sketches lent perspective to children's progress or lack of progress. The experience brought home to me the value of recording children's growth in reading and writing.

TWO STEPS FORWARD . . .

Eleven-year-old Curtis evokes a picture of his newly painted room:

> I can't believe I'm so lucky. This morning I opened my eyes and I thought I was in heaven . . .

Crystal, in fifth grade, grapples with her first attempt at mystery writing:

> "My mom lost her gold ring. She was so busy looking for that dumb ring that she didn't even have time for me. She didn't cook me dinner. Some mother she is," said Kristen in a mad voice.

Crystal continues:

> Liza was surprised to hear Kristen talk like that. She said,
> "Maybe that ring is important."
> "Well, if it was important she could have ordered dinner,"
> explained Kirsten with tears running down her cheeks.

Curtis' words of wonderment and Crystal's thinly veiled autobiography were inspired, in the sense that the words that flowed spontaneously from the children's pens succeeded in capturing the depth and flavor of their experiences.

Thomas Edison, however, observed that genius is only 1% inspiration and 99% perspiration. Perspiration, for writers, is tied up with the thoughtful shaping and reshaping of their writing. This brings both style and content closer and closer to expressing what it is the writers mean to convey.

. . . AND ONE STEP BACK

Twelve-year-old Shelley describes a party in honor of her great-aunt:

> I went to my great-aunt's party at my church. She was 90.
> Everybody danced. We ate a lot of food. Then we went
> home.

When I reacted with amazement that her great-aunt was ninety years old, Shelley burst out, "You should have seen her dance! When the music started playing, she got up and started dancing just like everybody else. We were all in a circle, and everybody was clapping. I was getting ready to cry."

As Shelley's words came tumbling out, I jotted them down. She listened as I read first the written, then the oral version of her story. Reluctantly, she admitted that the second account was more vivid.

I asked Shelley if she could start with the sentence, "You should have seen her dance!" and go on from there. Slowly she shook her head "no." I reminded her that when a writer tells a story with a great deal of feeling, as she had, those feelings come through to the reader. She did not respond. I named other resource room children who had elderly relatives of their own, and who might be touched by her experience. Shelley's final words were, "Maybe tomorrow . . ."

A WRITING STANDSTILL

The group log, individual logs, and essays attest to the progress of one group of children in spelling, language, and writing fluency. Children wrote with varying degrees of care and independence. Occasional pieces showed a grasp of genre, a developed ear for language, and the beginnings of competence in handling dialogue, multiple characters, and interwoven story lines. Several stories sustained the attention of both authors and readers through pages and even chapters.

Yet these pieces of writing remained islands of achievement tied to bursts of enthusiasm. Once their words were on the page, Curtis and Crystal were as far from exercising the craft of writing as was Shelley, with her unwillingness to make the effort required to put her story on paper.

I was faced with a dilemma. On the one hand, my notes reminded me that Curtis, for example, had been the first to begin to write reflectively, pausing to search for the words he needed. He had been the first to consider, with guidance, ways in which the form of his writing furthered the content. Curtis had moved into writing independently in the spring of fifth grade. I looked forward to the following September, eager to pick up where we had left off. I wondered where Curtis' writing would take him, and about my own ability to perceive his needs as an author and respond to them.

But instead of gathering strength, the promise of Curtis' earlier achievements faded into mediocrity. The same was true of the other children. It was as if they had lost whatever drive they had had to use writing to ponder and express the real concerns of their lives. As often as not, my help continued to be needed in all aspects of the writing process: coming up with an idea, narrowing it down and finding a focus, expanding and developing a topic. Children needed continuous encouragement to read their work to make sure that it conveyed what they had intended to say. This involved reading with an awareness of content, grammar, syntax, and legibility. In addition, it often fell on me to keep the sparkle of children's spontaneous oral language alive in their writing.

TRYING TO UNDERSTAND

I wonder to what degree factors related to the resource room setting may have affected children's attitudes toward writing.

Because the children had been so far below the level of their mainstreamed classes, I had devoted two years to developing basic skills. During those years, I closed my eyes to classroom-related needs and concentrated solely on reading and writing. Satisfying gains in both areas occurred during that time.

By then, a number of children were about to enter sixth grade. I felt responsible for helping them apply their basic skills to the work of their classes. This represented a fundamental change in resource room focus. Thoughtful writing takes time. The resource room period is short. My current goal did not permit the luxury of being able to focus exclusively on one area. Writing, like reading, had to fit the constraints imposed by the competing demands on resource room time. Perhaps it was not realistic to expect children to explore their lives in depth through writing, while telescoping the amount of time and attention devoted to writing in the resource room itself.

In addition, the absence of fellow-authors in all stages of the writing process left me as the main source of ideas, insights, and standards. In spite of wishing to share my experience as a writer among writers, this cast me in the role of authority and provoked resistance in several children.

These factors, along with my own relatively limited experience in helping children gather and expand on impressions related to their own lives, may have affected the development of my children as writers.

At the same time, no teaching can achieve results without the active participation of the learner. As the children became more competent writers, I felt that they were capable of taking on a greater share of responsibility for some of these functions. It seemed to me that writing with care, attention, and greater independence was no longer a question of ability, but of interest and desire. At a Writing Project conference in October 1993, Lucy Calkins spoke of the yearning to make writing better as being so important to the writing process. She quoted young children who already approach writing expecting it to be "so big," expecting it to "mean."

My recent experience had left me with the feeling that, for a variety of reasons, I had not succeeded in bringing this group of children to the point of combining proven ability with a commitment to do their best. "Maybe tomorrow . . ." expressed the doubt and uncertainty that lingered inside me for several years.

A SECOND CHANCE

Because basic language is a given for most school-age children, writers' workshops are free to focus on the depth, power, and beauty of the writing itself. The work of many of the young authors represented in whole language literature and conferences filled me with pleasure and awe. However, I came to realize that my longing to see this level of writing in the resource room had engendered unrealistic expectations for a group of children still in the process of overcoming language deficits.

Fellow authors and a ready audience are primary ingredients of writers' workshops. The resource room, on the other hand, is an optimal setting in which to help children express themselves in the language they already have, while offering them the skills needed for further development. In the resource room, the seeds of good writing can be planted, eventually to come to fruition in the classroom setting. Acknowledging the partnership between classroom and resource room reduced the tension which had accompanied my assuming responsibility for the entire process. The Writing Project's shift in emphasis from revision to writers' notebooks (Calkins 1991) also helped me rethink the process of fostering children's growth as writers.

As time went on, I decided to revive the idea of a collective log with a new group of children. Unlike the first group, these children ran the gamut from first grade through fifth, with a corresponding range of writing abilities. The original log had given pleasure to all participants. At the same time, I recalled the effort required to help the children generate ideas and put them down on paper. This, along with my mixed feelings regarding the quality and consistency of children's writing as they grew older, made me somewhat apprehensive. Nevertheless, I taped up a long strip of paper for each of us and lettered a brightly colored "Monday" on each sheet in preparation for the coming week.

The log took off in an unremarkable way. No one objected strenuously, but no one was particularly enthusiastic either. The children seemed to accept it as another class or resource room "have to," but without much seeing the point.

Within two or three weeks, I sensed a change. Children began to read one another's stories with real interest. Several children approached Douglas to ascertain, with a mixture of fearfulness and curiosity, why he wanted "to run away from home." He had left us hanging, unwilling to write more. At their urging, Douglas consented to write the sequel the next day: "When I ask my mother if I can have a drink, she says no."

Douglas, in turn, stood in front of Robert's latest news:

My baby brother is the first one to work at 9 or 10 months. When I showed the baby how to walk my mother ran to the couch. She said "The baby's walking! wow!"

"That's exciting," Douglas commented matter-of-factly. Coming from a child for whom social interaction was not yet easy or natural, this meant a lot.

Cathy took up her pencil to write about her dream. She got as far as "Yesterday . . ." She was not quite satisfied with the word. "Not 'yester . . . day,' " she mused; "I mean . . . yester-night!" She chuckled as she wrote that yesternight she had had the strangest dream. She was in her aunt's house:

They changed the house around and I do mean they changed it around. We were on the ceiling.

Cathy continued that her cousin had brought her a spider that turned into a hanger as she reached for it. "And, that's where it ends."

Some days, the children's stories flowed at length. At other times, a few sentences were all they needed:

Today I have to take my pill. It tastes like I am licking a dirty rug.

Cathy

Ms. Stelling's Tape
Ms. Stelling's tape looks like a baby carriage, right? When you put the tape standing up, you look at it very carefuly, and it looks like a baby carriage.

Emily

I was grateful for this log. In comparison with my experience of the past, I felt much more relaxed. The children, from the oldest to the youngest, were writing relatively freely and with enthusiasm, and I was enjoying their efforts. For all of us, this log was part of an ongoing learning experience. This time, my feeling was one of hope.

BEHIND THE SCENES

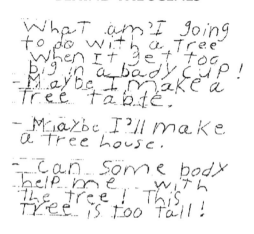

Finished pieces of writing such as Douglas' "tree" story, even when they contain uncorrected errors, do not convey the nature or extent of support needed by young deaf and hard-of-hearing children before they can achieve a degree of independence in writing. A session with Douglas, recorded verbatim, makes this process explicit.

Ms. S.: What's been happening while I was on jury duty?
D.: We did a lot of different things.
Ms. S.: Tell me.
D.: We learned about water germinate.
Ms. S.: You learned about seeds germinating!
D.: In science, you know, we had this red thing, and you can see the roots . . . *Douglas broke off, paused for a moment, then burst out with a humorous but heartfelt,* What am I going to do with the tree if it gets too big for the cup!
Ms. S.: You could start with that sentence! Could you say it again? *Douglas repeated the sentence and began to*

	write: What I. . . . *He stopped, having lost his thought.*
Ms. S.:	Listen, Douglas : What am I going to do with the tree . . . *I took out a piece of scrap paper for spelling attempts. Douglas wrote: What am I going to do with a tree?*
Ms. S.:	Remember you had more? *Douglas nodded. I prompted him.*
Ms. S.:	What am I going to do with the tree . . .
D.:	. . .when it gets too big for the cup. *He was about to write.*
Ms. S.:	Take away the question mark. When you finish writing, you can put it back at the end of the question. *Douglas complied, then went ahead willingly and completed his opening sentence, slightly altered. He was ready to call it a day. I pretended not to notice.*
Ms. S.:	Now you can go back and explain what you're talking about. Remember you told me what you were talking about?
D.:	I got more ideas. He wrote: *Maybe I'll make a Tree.* . . . *I eyed the word Tree in mock horror. Douglas started erasing furiously, his glance darting to the doorway.* Don't let the capital-letter police come, *he giggled. This was a joke from his days of scrambling upper and lower case letters. He continued, moving on to the word "tabel." He paused, then erased, declining my offer of scrap paper. I got it. He wrote "talbe," then "table." Douglas was using dashes to make a list, as he had seen me do in his resource room notebook. He continued writing: maybe . . .*
Ms. S.:	You're starting a new sentence. Period, capital. *Douglas changed the lower case to a capital. He wrote: Maybe I . . .*
Ms. S.:	Maybe I'll . . . In the future.
D.:	Is future real?
Ms. S.:	Sometimes it's real, sometimes it's imaginary. *Douglas continued:* . . . *build a tree houses. I pointed out that "a" is singular, "houses" plural, and explained that they needed to agree. Douglas decided he meant "a tree house." I mentioned the need for a period at the end of the sentence.*
D.:	I know. That's what I was going to write. *He resumed writing on his own:* "Can somebody help m. . . . *He lost concentration.*

> Ms.S. :   You're doing fine, Douglas. *He picked up where he left off: . . me with the tree? Douglas looked up, suddenly amused.*
>
> D.:   Oh, I got another sentence.
>
> Ms.S. :   What? *Douglas printed triumphantly: This tree is too tall!*

SUMMARY

Inspired by a lima bean, Douglas' five-sentence tour de force represented a leap forward for this eight-and-one-half-year-old writer. Douglas' language and behavioral difficulties related to the delayed diagnosis of his severe hearing loss are described at length in Chapters 18 and 21. By the end of second grade, when this story was written, Douglas had made a start in acquiring basic skills in a number of areas.

With Douglas, as with every child, it is necessary to choose what to address and what to let pass in any learning situation. During the writing of this story, Douglas was making the transition from primary paper to regular lined paper. His handwriting, while not perfect, was clear enough to be legible, and he was forming his letters with relative ease. Douglas tended to lean his head on his hand, leaving himself without a hand to keep the paper from shifting. I refrained from making an issue of it.

In writing about language development, Boothroyd (1988) outlines goals that "constitute a hierarchy in that a certain amount of success at one level is a prerequisite for progress at the next level." Boothroyd makes the point that, because these goals are also mutually dependent, every interaction between teacher and child should be designed to facilitate progress toward several goals at once. Paradoxically, "attainment of a given goal serves to reinforce its own prerequisites" (p. 74).

The evolution of Douglas' "tree story" illustrates the interdependence among grammar, punctuation, content, and general knowledge in the writing process. As he wrote, I drew to his attention several semi-familiar concepts. Seeds germinate, not water. Question marks belong at the end of a question, not in the middle. Capital letters have reasons for being, and are not to be used randomly. Periods are needed to signal the ends of sentences.

New to Douglas was the deliberate use of "I will" or "I'll" to denote future. Though he was acquainted with the concept of singular and plural, we had never talked about noun-verb agreement before.

This quantity of information—and interruptions—seemed sufficient. More would have felt like overload. Knowing this, I let go of several opportunities for correcting language and punctuation: "am' I." "When It get; bady." "and Maybe I make . . ." The fact that Douglas was cheerfully self-motivated, writing with a high degree of animation and independence, able to tolerate a teaching-learning partnership, and experiencing pleasure in the process was too precious to risk disturbing by overemphasizing accuracy. Opportunities for language development would continue to present themselves.

A SUPPORTIVE PRESENCE

My support of Douglas as he composed his story took several forms. I provided the opportunity for conversation to develop. I captured for him the moment at which fact and feeling combined to raise his narrative to a new level of aliveness. I introduced several grammatical concepts and reinforced others. Most important, I encouraged Douglas to tell me what he was about to write. I could then save him from frustration by keeping him on track in a way that he was not yet able to do for himself. Imperfections notwithstanding, Douglas produced four out of five vivid and cogent sentences with a minimum of overt intervention on my part. In contrast, Douglas' independent writing from the same period displays little of the clarity and coherence of stories created in the resource room with the teacher in close proximity, even when relatively little guidance was being offered. The following piece was written in the classroom and later corrected by the teacher.

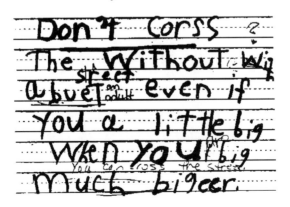

"What am I going to do with a tree when it get too big in a bady [*sic*] cup?" and " . . . even if you a little big when you big much bigeer" are both aspects of Douglas' writing ability at this moment. The difference in quality suggests that the resource room teacher's presence has an effect beyond preventing and correcting errors. By entering into a collaborative relationship, the teacher enhances by his or her very presence the tenuous abilities of a child such as Douglas who is struggling to set down his thoughts in writing. Even silent collaboration enables children to bring their focus and abilities to bear on the task at hand. In contrast, the multifaceted challenge of writing several sentences becomes overwhelming in the less structured classroom setting.

DOUGLAS: A SEQUEL

The input that Douglas required in order to produce a seemingly simple story is not an isolated phenomenon. Every young deaf or hard-of-hearing resource room child without exception has needed this kind of support for at least several years. A number of writing samples throughout the book were written by children who had reached the point of being able to write independently. Unless otherwise indicated, it should be understood that most pieces of writing were accompanied by some degree of collaboration similar to that which made Douglas' story possible.

Douglas produced his "tree story" in the spring of second grade. Half a year later, he came into the resource room, saw paper for the group log on the table, reached for a pencil, and wrote:

> My cub scout master gave me a box it had wood, nails and plastic wheel To make a car. Tonight I'm going To have a derby race. My derby car Name is Champion wildcat. IF I win I get a Trophy and a merit badge. I hope I win.

As he wrote, Douglas asked for help with the spelling of *derby, trophy,* and *badge.* I reminded him of several familiar phonics concepts and rules: trophy uses the alternate spelling of /f/; /long e/ at the end of *trophy* and *derby* is spelled *y*; /j/ after a vowel at the end of a word is likely to be spelled *dge.* Douglas applied this information without losing momentum. He was pleased with himself when he looked up to let me know he had finished.

I was elated at Douglas' first substantial piece of independent writing. These six colorful, coherent sentences signaled to me that our work had had a beneficial effect on Douglas' skills, which in turn influenced his attitude toward writing. I felt optimistic that this little paragraph would mark the beginning of a new level of writing for Douglas.

In fact, however, Douglas' moment of success was eclipsed by interrelated emotional and learning needs (for a more complete picture of Douglas as a learner, see Chapter 18). In the six remaining months of third grade, Douglas never equalled this achievement. Perhaps its very success was intimidating to him in some way. Hopefully, Douglas' slowly growing body of skills and accomplishments will one day help him move past his multifaceted resistance to learning.

LEARNING TO EDIT

Today when I went down stairs the bus left me. I saw the back of my bus leve I thogth that was my bus but I wanted to make sure. So I waited a littel longer. When I relies that was my bus I started to cry becuase I missed it I just started to walk to school.

Emily wrote "The Young Lady Who Missed the Bus" in the middle of fourth grade. Her days of needing a block tower to help her stretch an idea to three sentences were behind her. She no longer required squares of colored felt to help her retain her thoughts long enough to get them down on paper. Slowly, Emily had begun to relate her experiences in vivid and heartfelt pieces of writing.

I had shied away from drawing Emily's attention to grammar, punctuation, and spelling. In view of her earlier difficulties, I held my breath, not daring to disturb this still-tentative ability. For months, though, Emily had been coming into the resource room with stories she was bursting to tell. The ideas were her own, and she wrote confidently and with ease. Her writing had shape, coherence, and vitality.

For the first time, I sensed that Emily might be ready to stand back from her work and view it with a critical eye without damage to the flow and spontaneity of her writing. I began by explaining that the process of editing is not a sign of inadequate writing, but something that authors do to make sure their writing says what they mean it to say. I showed Emily a page from the computer printout of the manuscript of this book. Next I showed her the typewritten page that had preceded it, with its numerous corrections of all kinds. This was followed by several cut and taped hand-written pages, also heavily corrected. Finally, I brought out the original version, still in the composition notebook I carried with me wherever I went. These pages were so full of crossing out and rewording as to be indecipherable.

Bringing Emily's dyslexic spelling to her attention would be of little value until we could offer her a path to more accurate spelling. Like her language, Emily's spelling was improving with maturation and experience. Because of Emily's difficulties with auditory perception, many of the remaining errors were beyond her ability to correct at this point. Although the freshness of Emily's writing was a source of pleasure to all, it was difficult to convince her that editing did not have a negative connotation. Fortunately, this situation proved to be easily reversed by a trip to the nearest stationery store to select an editing pen in the color of her choice. With her turquoise pen in her pocket, Emily could hardly wait to begin editing.

At our next session, Emily watched as I turned an index card into an "Editing Checklist."

In selecting these items, I reasoned that periods seemed basic to good writing, and would make it possible to examine one sentence at a time. Subordinate clauses seemed to cry out for commas. I included them in spite of the lack of success I had experienced in trying to give children the tools of editing in the past. Last, I added spelling. My thinking was to have Emily point out any words she thought might be misspelled. I did not expect her to be able to correct most of them on her own, and had little idea to what extent she would be able to spot her own errors.

Emily surprised me on all three counts. She easily located the ends of her sentences. From that day on, she consistently ended her sentences with periods as she wrote. That part of the checklist became superfluous almost immediately. Using commas to signal a natural pause also made sense to Emily's ear, and she had no further problem with that aspect of writing. I could not have predicted this initial success in the area of editing.

Spelling provided another surprise. Emily was almost totally accurate in identifying misspelled words. Some she was able to correct on her own. Others reflected her still-weak auditory-visual grasp of vowels and diphthongs. For the first time, Emily began to monitor her own spelling as she wrote. While not always accurate or consistent, this conscious attention to her own writing without loss of spontaneity was a landmark for a child who had been unable to relate even two consecutive sentences about any event in her life only a few years earlier.

THE "SUNFLOWER STATE": A REPORT

"I'm so lucky I chose Kansas . . ." glowed Curtis, halfway through his first nonfiction writing project. He had come into the resource room ten days earlier, announcing that every child in his fifth-grade class had been assigned a report on a state. At age ten, Curtis barely understood the concept of "state," and had never heard of Kansas. Forging a connection between this boy and his topic was likely to be difficult.

The opportunity came along more easily than I had anticipated. As we opened an atlas together, I noticed that Kansas was perfectly rectangular except for a wiggly upper right-hand corner. Curtis was fascinated by this apparently odd configuration. By the time we identified the wiggle as the Missouri River, Curtis was bursting with enthusiasm for his adopted state.

The boundaries of Kansas led to an understanding of its terrain. Farming and industry made sense in light of this knowledge. Relating familiar children's books such as *The Wizard of Oz* (Baum 1988) and *Little House on the Prairie* (Wilder 1981) to what Curtis was learning made factual reading more personal.

Once Curtis had amassed some basic information, we headed several sheets of paper with key words such as "geography" and "products." Curtis jotted down relevant information by topic as we went along. This made it easier when the time came to organize and develop what he had learned. Discovering that Kansas was the "Sunflower State" gave Curtis the opportunity to combine knowledge and artistic ability into an attractive report cover.

PREREQUISITES TO NONFICTION WRITING

The following section is based on Graves (1989).

Nonfiction writing has its roots in young children's expressive language. Children build language and cognitive skills basic to report-writing as they expand one-sentence stories about incidents and events in their lives, describe how they work and learn (for example the process of cutting something out), and interpret data from class-made graphs. Learning to recognize dual points of view related to everyday controversies enables children to write one-sentence opinions supported by one or two facts as early as first grade. Observing, recording, and reviewing data leads to an awareness of the processes that take place around us.

Graves recommends that children approach report-writing by:

- making a list of things they know how to do, or areas of knowledge they feel they already know something about;
- selecting a topic;
- making a web;
- focusing on one aspect of the web and formulating questions about it;
- finding appropriate reading material; and
- making notes from reading.

Discussing each phase of report-writing with a partner clarifies the process and helps children solidify their knowledge of content. It is this knowledge that gives children the sense of

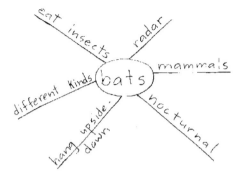

authority that allows their own voices to emerge in their writing. The cycle of discussion, reading, and taking notes repeats itself until children are ready to organize their information and begin writing.

NONFICTION WRITING AND THE LANGUAGE-DELAYED CHILD

Curtis' report evolved in a much different way. Because Curtis had no prior interest or knowledge to bring to this project, I had to help create both. Because he could not read independently at the required level, I needed to guide him in his selection of books, determine what passages to read, and provide assistance as he read. Because writing of any kind was still difficult for Curtis, the added challenge of organizing totally unfamiliar material was beyond his ability. Providing a structured method of recording information became my responsibility.

Curtis' report was successful in that he was able to carry out a class assignment with interest and enthusiasm. It was less than successful in that a high proportion of input from me was crucial to every aspect of his work. Graves notes that the teachers's task is to keep alive a "sense of awe and wonder" (p. 99) and to offer feedback as to where children stand in the writing process. My contribution to Curtis' project needed to be far more extensive.

Reading even simplified material, taking notes, and developing a piece of connected writing are beyond the ability of children who are still in the process of acquiring basic language. At age ten, Curtis was close to having attained this basic language competence along with the background knowledge that would enable him to feel some measure of expertise in areas of personal interest. Just as he was becoming more capable of understanding and using everyday language, Curtis found himself faced with a volume of unfamiliar vocabulary. Hearing children, who over-hear language that goes on around them, are likely to be at least superficially acquainted with curriculum-related vocabulary. Children with impaired hearing are more limited in their expo-sure to language. This was Curtis' first encounter with such words as *boundaries, agriculture, industry*, and *terrain*. This made the reading and writing related to his report particularly difficult.

Going back to picture books helped a group of fairly liter-ate fifth graders develop an awareness of authors, illustrators, and themes (Chapter 12). It would be possible and profitable, once children have gained an adequate language foundation, to go back and develop the sequence of skills basic to nonfiction writing. Unlike picture books, which were used in an incidental way, this process would need to become the focus of resource room learning for an extended period of time. The dilemma, for me, has been that I have felt reluctant to sacrifice academic sup-port just as children are beginning to move toward fuller partici-pation in their mainstream classes.

As a result, children have been faced with the demands of report writing without having acquired the skills and strategies needed to develop a piece of nonfiction writing comfortably and independently. Whether or not to persevere with report writing has depended on the extent to which a child is able to move beyond the assistance that is initially required.

The guidance John received with his research on pandas (see Chapter 2) did not bring him closer to independence in any aspect of his writing. Postponing report writing while concentrat-ing on basic skills was clearly a more beneficial use of resource room time. In contrast, Curtis' sustained interest, combined with his ability to take over some of the reading and writing, indicated that our work on Kansas was a true partnership. I believed that Curtis was integrating some of what he was learning, and would be able to apply it to future projects. This made it worthwhile to undertake assignments of this nature in spite of the amount of di-rection required.

Along with specific skills, two factors bring children closer to being able to attempt nonfiction writing. The first is ongoing language development. The second is the systematic acquisition of general knowledge.

Chapter 16

The Quest for Knowledge

Once children develop basic vocabulary and language skills and are reasonably oriented in their family and school lives, something has to begin the process of broadening their acquaintance with the world. The four-year old who walks along the street asking, "Daddy, did dinosaurs live in prehistoric times?" has already digested and integrated important scientific and historical concepts. A deaf or hard-of-hearing child of seven, eight, or even nine may be just beginning to acquire this kind of knowledge.

In a home or other family setting, information can be imparted in a casual and natural way as opportunities arise. The resource room is a more limited environment. While we need to be alert to opportunities, we cannot sit back and wait for them to come along. We have to arrange for them to present themselves in a world of knowledge so vast and so varied that figuring out how and where to begin is sometimes overwhelming.

AWARENESS OF THE WORLD: A BEGINNING

Two things have helped. The first was the realization that one starting point is as good as another. Any piece of knowledge leads to a second, which leads to a third. By that time, it is already possible to point out connections and begin to make associations. In effect, two threads emerge simultaneously: the amassing of information of all kinds; and the thinking skills that bring meaning and order to what would otherwise remain an assortment of unrelated facts.

The second helpful discovery has been learning to make the acquisition of information systematic and tangible. This has taken various forms.

The "Information Notebook"

What worked for eight-year-old Dahlia and for several children after her was an "information notebook." Recording facts and concepts gave our work in this area a shape and a coherence that had been lacking. The process of entering new information in a clear and official way was compelling in itself. It was then easy to leaf through the pages and converse about previously learned material.

Sometimes quickly, sometimes more slowly, Dahlia gained ease and familiarity with old concepts and with the language needed to discuss them. As this happened, we turned our attention to newer material.

Information came from various sources: reading, classwork, and casual conversation. The following activities illustrate two possible uses of the information notebook. In the first, the notebook was used to clarify the meaning of "sunrise" without interrupting the flow of the story from which it came. For this reason, the discussion was brief and self-contained, with no related ideas growing out of it.

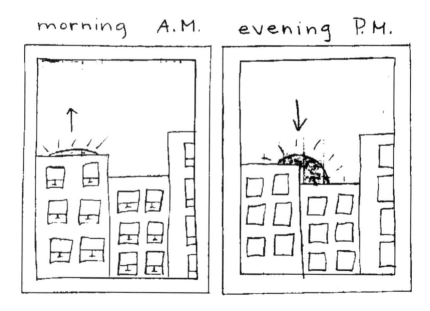

The second activity originated with map work on the five boroughs of New York City. From there we went on to identify each continent, beginning with North America, on a wooden world map puzzle. We discussed one continent at a time while coloring it in on an outline map. We expanded on this knowledge by linking familiar people, places, animals, clothing, and means of transportation to each continent. The process of reinforcing what Dahlia had begun to learn, then adding and integrating new material, formed part of every resource room session for several weeks.

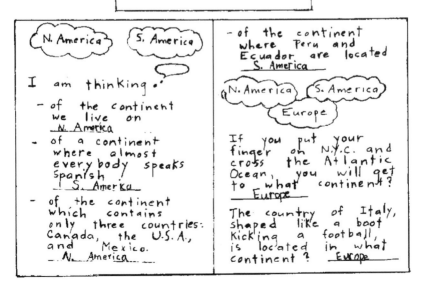

If you are in Europe and you travel south, you will come to the continent of <u>Africa</u>.

<u>Africa</u> has many countries, all squooshed together.

<u>North America</u> is different. It has only three countries.

We know someone who comes from Asia: <u>Tony</u> !

Asia has three big countries (and

Some smaller countries):
1. China
2. Russia
3. Japan

Black and white panda bears live in <u>China</u> .

Pandas eat bamboo.

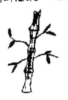

Bamboo grows only in the mountains in China.

If you are in Asia and you travel south, you get to what continent ? <u>Australia</u>

If you go to Australia, you'll hear people speaking English

You'll see some animals that are found only in Australia. For example:

1. Kangaroo
2. Koala bear

Some continents have many countries all crowded together. For instance, <u>Africa</u> and <u>Europe</u> .

But Australia has only <u>one</u> country

Continent: <u>Australia</u>
Country: <u>Australia</u>

One continent is all the way south. It's called <u>Antarctica</u> .

If you live in N.Y.C. and want to travel to Italy, you have to cross what body of water ? <u>Atlantic ocean</u>

What is the biggest continent ? <u>Asia</u>

Asia is right next to what other continent ? <u>Europe</u>

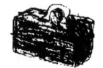

Traveling Time

If you want to get from North America to Europe, how could you travel ?

You can travel by boat because you have to cross the Atlantic Ocean.

Three ways of traveling:

1.) By land (by car, By school bus, By train, By bus)

2.) By sea (. by boat, By ship)

3.) By air (By airplane)

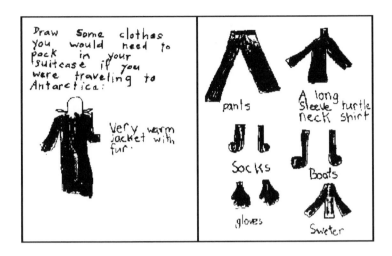

To Expand or Not to Expand: A Question

Any concept can engender an array of new ideas, all of which can lead in fascinating directions. There is nothing in the concept of "sunrise-sunset" that is inherently less interesting or less worthy of being developed than the naming of the continents. We could have explored day and night in different parts of the world, the rotation of the earth, nocturnal animals, or occupations that entail working at night.

At times, a child's own interests lead naturally to activities designed to reinforce his or her knowledge and expand on it. At times, teacher-initiated activities are needed in order to create awareness where none existed before. Dahlia had neither interest nor understanding to bring to our introductory work on the continents. Both developed as we built a foundation of knowledge by linking familiar concepts to new geographical information. The decision whether to touch on a concept briefly, explore it more fully, or bypass it altogether is also influenced by the child's level, the amount of time available, and the relative importance of a given topic to the learning needs of a child at that moment.

Whether brief or thorough, every encounter that sparks children's interest furthers our goal of broadening their understanding of the world.

Meeting the World Through Art

I recently made a small beginning on a project I had been envisioning for some time. I have wanted to set up a lending library of postcard reproductions from the Metropolitan Museum of Art and other museums. My thought is to provide each child with a 4″ x 6″ standing frame to keep at home. Children would select and borrow postcards from our collection, and live with those works of art until ready to exchange them for others.

One day I took the first step and bought two or three dozen postcards representing a range of time periods, cultures, artists, and styles. I put them in a box and divided them according to historical periods. I labeled the back of each postcard with simple identifying information.

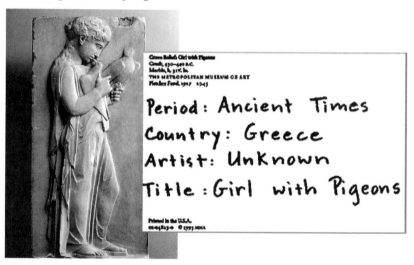

Period: Ancient Times
Country: Greece
Artist: Unknown
Title: Girl with Pigeons

The Metropolitan Museum of Art, Fletcher Fund, 1927. (27.45).

This happened toward the end of the school year. Since I had not yet bought frames, the postcards stayed in school. Several children and I spent a leisurely afternoon looking through our "art collection." The children were entranced by the beautiful array of vases, statues, frescoes, reliefs, drawings, and paintings. Ten-year-old John was motivated to ask his father to take him to the museum to see the exhibit of ancient Greek sculpture. He came in after the weekend with his own postcard of "Girl with Pigeons," which had been his favorite.

Though my experience with an art lending library is still limited, I sense that it has tremendous potential as a means of:

- expanding children's knowledge of history and geography;
- acquainting children with art, artists, and museums; and
- offering children an opportunity to develop an appreciation of art of all kinds.

Children, like adults, have the capacity to be delighted, even moved by works of art. They can learn to love and appreciate beauty and creativity while beginning to discover their own tastes and leanings. Introducing children to art can add interest and meaning to their lives.

Timelines

"In ancient times . . ."
"During the Middle Ages . . ."
"By the end of the Renaissance . . ."
"In pioneer days . . ."
"Before modern times . . ."
"Many centuries ago . . ."

Hearing children absorb the language of time relationships. These concepts gradually become part of their growing comprehension and ability to express themselves.

Children who are deaf and hard of hearing need help to take in and make sense out of the patchwork of information that comes to them in bits and pieces as they advance through the grades. Once the underlying language concepts have meaning, the people and events of history have a chance of falling into place.

Using a timeline has been a valuable way of making abstract concepts and relationships visible and comprehensible. A timeline gives perspective to historical figures and events. It places them in relation to one another in a way that is visible and concrete. A timeline serves as a taking-off point for discussion appropriate to each child's level and experience. It creates the opportunity for time concepts and relationships to be introduced and reinforced.

Variation I

I have experimented with two kinds of timelines. The first was a row of pieces of oaktag headed "Prehistoric Times, Ancient Times, Middle Ages . . ." Each period was represented by two postcards or drawings. We used the timeline in a casual and informal way to locate events from history and children's literature as they came up.

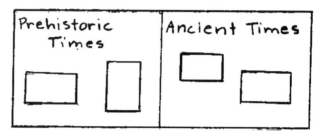

That year, the resource room included a group of older children who had progressed through the grades together. The children had done a great deal of reading and had a fair acquaintance with children's literature. However, their fund of factual information was extremely limited. The timeline provided a means of moving from the relatively familiar world of children's stories to the less known realm of real-life events through the ages.

It would be exciting and worthwhile to build an entire curriculum around a timeline. This has not been possible because of the many issues that need to be addressed in the resource room. The timeline remained in the background, a valuable ally in deepening children's understanding. When twelve-year-old Crystal read a short story about a farm woman who stood her ground against her husband (Freeman 1967), we searched the story for clues that would place it in history. We located it along the timeline using knowledge gained from previous discussions.

Books were sometimes chosen to introduce unfamiliar time periods. *The Microscope* (Kunin 1986) captured the flavor of the Renaissance by its description of van Leeuwenhoek's fascination with magnification. From then on, we were able to relate other Renaissance discoveries and inventions to this common reference point.

Children also enjoyed hearing stories and biographical sketches from time periods with which they had some familiarity. They pieced together what they knew about clothing, transportation, inventions, events, and historical figures, both real and fictitious. They used this knowledge to place, for example, Sarah Noble and her wilderness journey in the context of colonial times.

The timeline was a useful learning tool for all the children. It was particularly meaningful to those children with a strong leaning toward history and science. Tom, now in sixth grade, had begun asking questions such as "How volcano born?" the moment he was able to put three words together. Because of his severe hearing loss and lack of exposure to English outside of school, Tom's language lagged far behind his ability and achievement in math and science. This was a source of frustration.

Perhaps for that reason, precision and order were very satisfying to Tom. The timeline enabled him to bring order to his growing knowledge of the world. Toward the end of the year, it became necessary to take the timeline down. It would have been best to do this with the children, but in the interest of efficiency I took it down myself. Sensing how much the timeline had meant to Tom, I folded it up and saved it for him. When he saw the empty wall, he flared up in anger until I offered him the bag to take home. The timeline had met a need in this child deeper than any I had originally foreseen.

Variation II

After this group of children graduated, a very different situation ensued. Several new children, already in the middle grades, entered the resource room program. They were close to being nonreaders. Their awareness of the world ranged from scanty to almost none. Basic reading skills took precedence over everything else.

Once the children were able to read with the slightest degree of fluency, we began to include informational material among our reading selections. Nine-year-old Cathy had barely begun to acquire the diverse knowledge that would one day enable her to appreciate the Valentine's Day romance of two Holocaust survivors (see pp. 98–100). After reading and listening to a picture biography of George Washington, Cathy said that she was "starting to be interested in learning about, you know . . . things." By this, Cathy meant real people and events. Her remark led me to think about what kind of timeline could help these young children acquire and consolidate knowledge at their levels.

I hung up a series of large sheets with headings. Next to them I taped up an envelope containing blank cards.

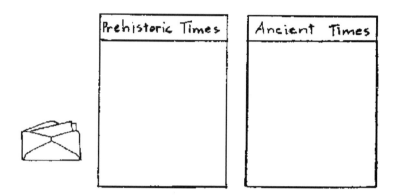

As we came across information that belonged to one historical period or another, children would take cards, jot down key words, and tape them up on the timeline. Sometimes children described what they had learned in two or three sentences. Newspaper photos of covered wagons on the Oregon Trail, drawings of constellations that guided runaway slaves to freedom, a shoebox loom we made to experience how weaving had been invented as far back as prehistoric times, a dollar bill with its portrait of the first president—all these made the timeline interesting and colorful. They formed a scaffold that helped each new piece of information fall more clearly into place. The web of information became increasingly rich and interrelated.

Information came along during reading, discussion, and even casual conversation. I chose books to read to and with the children, with the aim of introducing unfamiliar historical periods or building on previous knowledge. From *Living in Prehistoric Times* (Chisholm 1982), we became acquainted with mammoths, cave art, weaving, and early tools and weapons. *Children of Ancient Greece* (Wilson 1974) introduced us to togas, school life, architecture, and democracy.

Little by little, the children added to their fund of general knowledge. We observed threads that ran through more than one time period. The children began to perceive relationships and to be able to put them into words. Clothing through the ages was easy to compare and contrast. We talked about how clothes were made and by whom, what they were made of and why. Weaving, which dates back to earliest times, has continued to develop throughout the ages. We made a simple loom, did some weaving, and noticed how looms and weaving have changed with the passage of time.

Structure of Timeline

It was not so simple to decide how to name the various eras along each of the timelines. Historical periods can be subdivided. One era blends into another. The "Renaissance" applies to Europe, whereas colonial and pioneer days pertain to American history.

A timeline can compartmentalize history and culture in a neat but misleading way. I discovered it was possible to use the timeline to show that different ways of living occurred simultaneously. In some parts of the country, settlers built simple cabins. In others, towns grew up, and architecture and furnishings became much more ornate. All of this came under the umbrella of "colonial days."

At every opportunity we took note of the history and achievements of Africa and Asia, and related them to the basic timeline we were using.

Our use of timelines was based on children's developing interests and knowledge. Incorporating reading, writing, and projects of various kinds gave meaning to abstract concepts. Although they simplified history, timelines played a valuable role in helping children understand the world and their place in it.

Chapter 17

Personalizing Knowledge

As children grow, it becomes important to give them a clear understanding of their own hearing. In addition to incidental learning and discussion, several projects were developed in response to this need.

A school science fair was scheduled around the time that Curtis, Crystal, and Shelley were about to graduate. Curtis announced with great excitement that he was going to make a volcano. I reluctantly explained that making a volcano was more an art project than a science project; that a science project entails asking a question, figuring out a way to find the answer, and carrying it out.

Not having a scientific bent, I groped for an example. "For instance," I thought aloud, "suppose you wondered how useful FM units really are compared to hearing aids. You could set up an experiment to find that out." The minute the words were out, I became excited. I realized I could give these three children a parting gift so that they would start junior high school fully aware of the value of their FM units.

HEARING AIDS AND FM UNITS: A COMPARISON

Our educational audiologist guided me in setting up the project. The children marked off every three feet on the floor with masking tape. Their enthusiasm built as they backed out the door and progressed down the hallway, measuring and taping as they went. The three sixth graders, along with two younger children, then took turns testing one another. They used a word list consisting of equally accented compound words such as "hotdog," "mailman," and "baseball." An actual hearing test given in a soundproof booth would use monosyl-labic words, but these would have been too difficult to hear against the background noise of the schoolroom and corridor.

Two rounds of testing were done: the first with hearing aids, the second with FM units. The children needed to repeat three out of five words correctly in order to move back. The child whose turn it was to read from the word list kept a record of how far back his or her partner was able to move and still hear the words.

The results were dramatic. With hearing aids, children were generally unable to distinguish the words at all after eight feet. With the FM units, they could hear and discriminate words all the way out of the room and down the hall to a distance of 110 feet and more. This was true even with traffic between class-rooms and bathrooms, and classes passing through the hall.

Children recorded their results on a bar graph. Each child's ability to hear with hearing aids was represented by a short bar. In contrast, we needed to add on sheets and sheets of oaktag in order to accommodate the bars that represented hearing in noise and over distance with the FM units.

Language, writing, math, and science all came into play as the project developed. We took into account what kinds of in-formation visitors to the science fair would need in order to un-derstand what the project was about. The children made a chart describing the project, and another labeling and explaining the parts of a hearing aid and FM unit. They copied their audio-grams and were able to describe their hearing losses in terms of mild or moderate, severe or profound.

At the science fair, the children had an FM unit with micro-phone available for others to listen to. They also had a tray of "hands-on" items for children to handle. These items included hearing aid and FM batteries, battery testers, earmolds, cords, and the stethescope used for checking amplification devices. In addi-tion, they took turns demonstrating how to mix impression mate-rial and squirt it from a syringe to make an earmold.

The "hands-on" material and earmold demonstration made the exhibit a popular one with visitors to the fair. Two aspects of the project proved especially valuable to the resource room chil-dren themselves. The first was experiencing the undeniable ben-efit of the FM units. The second was the children's willingness, despite some initial reluctance, to display and explain their au-diograms in public, thus acknowledging that they accepted and felt comfortable sharing this aspect of who they are.

INVENTING AN AUDIOMETER

Curtis, Crystal, and Shelley were about to enter junior high school at the time of their science fair project. Over the years, even much younger children have expressed interest in the display of audiograms on the resource room wall. I have wondered how to convey this technical information in an understandable way. A makeshift "audiometer" helped solve the problem. It consisted of a 9" by 12" piece of oaktag labeled "audiometer," with an arrow denoting "decibels."

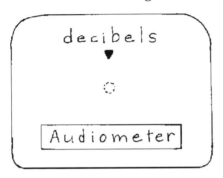

In the center we placed a $3^{1}/_{2}$" oaktag dial subdivided into decibels and labeled with the corresponding hearing losses. The designations were contrastingly colored for easy visibility:

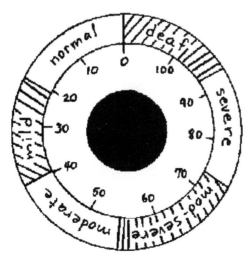

A two-pronged paper fastener attached the dial to the audiometer through a hole in the center of each. This allowed for easy turning. A plastic bottle cap was glued bottom down to the center of the dial, concealing the paper fastener. Children used this knob to rotate the dial through the various decibels and hearing levels.

UNDERSTANDING AUDIOGRAMS

Emily and Cathy, one in fourth grade and the other in fifth, had expressed curiosity about their audiograms. As soon as the audiometer was hung up, the girls took their audiograms down from the wall and colored the different hearing levels to correspond to the colors on the dial of the audiometer. The normal range was blue, the mild range green, and so on. We traced each child's hearing through the high, middle, and low frequencies. I gave each of the girls a mock hearing test, explaining that the audiologist had to turn the dial up to 30 dBHL (decibels Hearing Level), 40 dBHL, 50 dBHL or higher before they could hear the beeps.

In the days that followed, we repeated the process several times. To this information we added the knowledge that the girls' audiograms improve dramatically when they take the same test wearing their hearing aids or FM units. Robert and Douglas, both younger, enjoyed twirling the dial of the audiometer, but were less interested initially in an in-depth explanation.

A Demonstration Hearing Test

All resource room children have their hearing tested periodically. All of them are familiar with the process of putting on headphones and raising their hands when they hear the beeps. Our recent work had introduced basic concepts related to hearing loss. At this point, the audiologist serving our resource room program offered to cooperate in increasing the children's understanding of audiological testing.

Soon afterward, four children from second through fifth grade crowded into an audiological testing booth and began reading *Patrick Gets Hearing Aids* (Riski 1994). The children recognized themselves over and over in this story of a little rabbit with a newly diagnosed hearing loss. Several children nodded knowingly when Patrick turns up the volume of the television as his brother and sister cringe in the corners of the sofa. Douglas related to a picture of Patrick's classmates working on writing assignments while Patrick just scribbles, not having understood the teacher's directions.

The depiction of Patrick's hearing test is true to life in every detail, and includes an actual audiogram. Cathy's experience reading her own audiogram enabled her to interpret Patrick's. She described for us that Patrick had hearing in the mild range, dropping down to moderate, then to mod-severe. Cathy was justifiably pleased with herself.

The Hearing Test

Ear infections exert pressure on the eardrum. Hearing testing performed on a child with a middle ear infection may not be indicative of the child's hearing under normal circumstances. To ascertain that the children's eardrums were vibrating normally, the audiologist began by testing each child's middle ear with a tympanometer. She inserted a probe into the child's outer ear. The probe was connected to a computer, which emitted a printout (see p. 171).

One child at a time then went to the other side of the testing booth. The others stayed behind, watching the audiologist manipulate the volume dial and frequency button of the audiometer. All four children happened to have symmetrical hearing losses— nearly the same in both ears. Because time was limited, the audiologist tested each child's right ear only. Through the one-way mirror, the children witnessed one another's failure to respond, then uncertainty, then definite reaction as the audiologist increased the volume to the child's hearing level. They saw her obtain each child's hearing thresholds and record the results on an audiogram.

To make the experience an active one, the audiologist allowed the children to take turns testing her hearing. With my help, each child selected a low, middle, or high frequency. Starting at 35 dBHL, they decreased the volume and recorded the lowest volume at which the audiologist raised her hand. Even more thrilling was the opportunity to put on the audiologist's microphone and query, "Can you hear me?"

It had been a long morning. The sequence of activities had sustained the children's interest and attention. Time would tell how much each child had taken in. But, already, the experience had enriched their understanding and mine.

CO-AUTHORING A BOOK

The children had been exposed to a quantity of information during our hours in the testing booth. I wanted to help them make sense of their impressions and solidify their understanding. I decided that writing a booklet together would provide the opportunity we needed for questions and discussion.

As a starting point, I wrote a sequence of sentences outlining our experience. I cut the sentences apart and attached each one to the top of a blank page with a paper clip. As children came to the resource room, they read through these ten or twelve pages. Different children reacted to different sections. The booklet filled up as children formulated their thoughts aloud, then in writing. Many responses were spontaneous, and communicated in the children's own words. Children generally needed help to express their understanding of the more technical aspects of audiological testing. The concepts and language were difficult and unfamiliar, as they would be to any child or adult on first acquaintance.

Taking Shape

The quantity of writing clipped to the pages of our booklet grew daily. Children responded to my original sentences and to one another's. By the end of two or three weeks, we were ready to embark on the editing process. I rewrote my sentences neatly on blank pages. Children cut out and taped in their pieces of writing, while I added connecting words and sentences where needed. Emily appointed herself illustrator.

The finished booklet was 29 pages long. We came up with several possible titles, and combined the two favorite choices into *Children Who Have Hearing Aids: Understanding How We Hear*. The children listed everyone they wanted to receive a copy of the booklet. In addition to the children themselves, the list included our audiologists, a variety of teachers and administrators, as well as classroom, resource room, and school libraries.

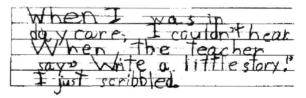

The first thing we did was to squeeze
inside the testing booth and read
"Patrick Gets Hearing Aids."

Douglas understood how Patrick felt:

When I was in
day care, I couldn't hear
When the teacher
says "write a little story,"
I just scribbled.

Emily describes having a tympanogram:

> Annette had this instrument and she had a litte computer. She put the instrument into your ear and the computer touches your ear. It gives you a sheet like this:

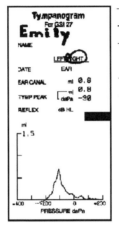

> The line looks like a mountain. And it means that your ear drum is OK

Emily noticed:

> Me and Patrick, has the same color of ear molds. When you put the pink stuff in your ear it feels cold.

Cathy knew how to read Patrick's audiogram:

> Patrick's hearing starts in the mild range, then drops down to mod-severe, then to severe.

Emily observed what the audiologist was doing:

> Annette was truning the knob back-
> and forth, to make it softer and
> louder.

Here is Cathy's reaction:

> It felt like it was my imagination
> because the beep sounds were low.

We changed places. Douglas and
Emily had their hearing tested
while Robert and Cathy watched.

Douglas

Emily

Robert had the same reaction as
Cathy:

> That happened to me too!
> I thought she made a beep but I
> didn't hear it that well. I raised my
> hand anyway.

Emily listened as hard as she could:

> I had to rase my hand when I heard the beep. They were loued, medium, and low.

Cathy kept her eye on the audiometer:

> I saw how it works and it was Interesting. There was a knob to change the volume. We press a button to change the frequency.

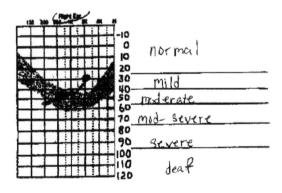

normal

mild

moderate

mod-severe

severe

deaf

Cathy: My hearing loss starts in the moderate ranges, then goes up to the mild range.

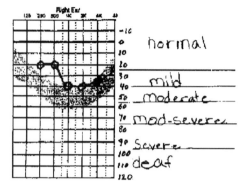

Robert: I have normal hearing in the lower frequencies. I have a mild hering loss in the higher frequencies.

It was Annette's turn for a hearing test. The children took turns being audiologists.

Emily recalls:

I put the headbard on my head, and the speaker near my lips. I asked "Can you hear me?" Annette said "I can hear you."

Each person chose a high, middle, or low frequency.

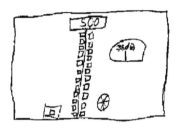

Emily went first.

I picked 500 H Z. That's a very low frequency.

Now we understand...

Emily:

When Someone talks to me and I took off my hearing aids, I can't hear what they said that well because I have a hearing loss. But when I put my hearing aids on, my hear is normal.

Cathy:

Now I know that people have different kinds of hearing loss. Even the four of us has different hearing losses.

Douglas:
I don't under stand
The inner ear and the
middle ear. The
Sound go in the outer
ear. It goes
Through The ear canal.

Robert:
When someone talks to you,
the sound goes into the ear
canal. Then it hits the ear
drum. The ear drum hits the
hammer and the hammer hits the
anvil, the sound slides in to your
inner-ear, then your brain.

Children Who Have Hearing Aids: Understanding How We Hear grew out of a first-hand experience of deep personal interest. Explanation, discussion, and the use of manipulative materials had prepared the children for active learning during the testing situation. The experience provided a rich source of material for integrated learning. It combined cognitive and affective learning. It integrated math, science, reading, and oral and written language. Seeing the making of a booklet through from start to finish served as a model for future undertakings, both cooperative and independent.

Chapter 18

Incorporating Phonics

Phonics instruction presents problems to children with limited hearing. Depending upon his or her hearing loss, a child may perceive some sounds normally, others not at all, and still others with varying degrees of distortion. Children's ability to discriminate speech sounds often develops considerably with auditory training. Nevertheless, learning to make letter-sound associations can be a major undertaking for a hearing-impaired child.

In addition, hearing loss reduces children's exposure to language. Systematic work in language development contributes to the growth of grammar, syntax, and vocabulary. Phonics instruction does not become feasible until a fair level of language has been achieved. Sounding out is of questionable value when word after word goes unrecognized because it falls outside the scope of a child's limited vocabulary.

For this reason, I have favored a language-oriented approach to reading, with phonics incidental and secondary. Despite this conviction, I found myself becoming increasingly concerned that even the reasonably good readers among the resource room children remained unable to decode many an unfamiliar word, or to write words that were not remembered visually. I began to feel uncomfortable with the knowledge that I was not helping children take the next step in reading and writing.

A DISCOVERY

Some approaches that have been developed for other populations can be adapted to the needs of deaf and hard-of-hearing children.

Children with reading and auditory processing problems associated with dyslexia have difficulty making sound-symbol connections. The Orton Gillingham approach to the teaching of reading and writing (Gillingham and Stillman 1965) is among the methods developed in response to the needs of such children. It is a highly structured, repetitive, multisensory approach that progresses from vowels and consonants to blends, diphthongs, and digraphs. Programs based on Orton Gillingham, such as Alphabetic Phonics, incorporate a pictorial association with each sound so that it becomes fixed in the child's eye and ear simultaneously.

These fundamental building blocks are interwoven and reinforced by means of a daily sequence of reading, spelling, and handwriting activities that involve children in looking, listening, vocalizing, and movement. Children learn to simplify the task of decoding by recognizing combinations of letters that produce a single sound, with the gradual introduction of prefixes and suffixes. From there they move on to basic formulas for syllable division that give children a tool for decoding words of any length.

Because many of the children with whom I work display classic signs of learning disability along with hearing loss, I decided to become familiar with the Orton Gillingham approach. At the same time, I was skeptical about its value for children who could not hear well enough to discriminate sounds accurately or produce them clearly. I also continued to have serious reservations about emphasizing phonics with children who barely had everyday words at their command.

In order to ascertain the benefits of such an approach for this particular population, I began incorporating it into my work with several children.

CATHY

In spite of her growth in language and general information, Cathy continued to show evidence of specific learning disabilities. She had difficulty grasping the connection between letters or combinations of letters and the sounds they represent. She also had difficulty perceiving the sequence of sounds within words. These weaknesses affected her ability to read and write. Cathy had been a nonreader when she entered the resource room program. She was about to repeat third grade, since she had not come close to working on third-grade level the year before. Her language was at a basic conversational level. In the course of two years of intensive instruction in a self-contained class for children with learning disabilities with additional resource room support, Cathy's language and reading had moved forward. Yet reading was still a struggle for her. I decided to attempt to give Cathy a foundation in phonics that could help her read more fluently and confidently.

A Breakthrough

Cathy's reading improved slowly but steadily with the help of the Orton Gillingham approach. One day, feeling the need to see visible signs of progress, I went straight to the sophisticated skill of syllable division (see pp. 127–128). Contrary to what I had feared, Cathy grasped this concept quickly and easily. Within a few days, she was decoding long unfamiliar words. She was thrilled with herself, and told me how proud her parents were of her ability to read her most recent vocabulary words.

This breakthrough clarified for me the relationship between the various elements of the Orton Gillingham method. Cathy had mastered a core of letter-sound associations with the help of the picture deck, which displayed a letter or combination of letters along with a picture clue on each card.

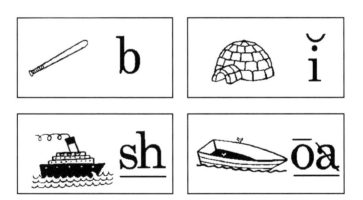

These associations had been reinforced by the reading deck, consisting of letters without pictures (Initial Reading Deck by Aylett R. Cox. Reproduced with permission from Educators Publishing Service, Cambridge, MA. Copyright 1971). Cathy had learned to blend sounds orally—first by imitation, then on her own. Oral blending provided a basis for visual blending, or the sounding out of sequences of letters.

"Coding" exercises gave Cathy practice drawing a box around frequently used suffixes, as well as underlining letter combinations that make a single sound, e.g., /sh/, /tch/, /oa/, /au/. These two multi-kinesthetic operations simplified the decoding process by leaving the base word clearly visible and drawing attention to familiar letter combinations.

<u>sh</u>ip

h<u>au</u>nt

c<u>oa</u>ch

bend[ing]

<u>ph</u>one[s]

Once Cathy could decode short words with ease, several strategies for dividing words into syllables enabled her to apply her growing knowledge of letter-sound associations to multi-syllabic words. A small number of spelling rules gave her a means of determining, for example, when to use /k/ or /ck/ at the end of a word, and when to double a final consonant before an ending. Daily spelling practice consisting of sounds in isolation, in words, and in sentences, reinforced sounds and rules as they were learned, and developed Cathy's ease and automaticity in writing.

A Structured Phonics Method in Perspective

When Cathy joined the resource room program, she had already repeated kindergarten and was about to repeat third grade. Cathy scored at a low second-grade level on evaluations of letter-word identification and oral comprehension. Receptive and expressive vocabulary were within the average range for her current grade level. She had difficulty supplying antonyms, using words to make associations ("What goes with milk?"), and describing ways in which items were similar or different. Cathy had difficulty reading unfamiliar words.

A writing sample ("the brid is sining in his kache") revealed Cathy's weakness in making sound-symbol associations, as well as her difficulty perceiving sounds in sequence. Both classroom teacher and evaluator noted difficulties in the areas of verbal reasoning and auditory association.

After repeating third grade with resource room support, Cathy scored in the 11th percentile on a cloze test that called heavily upon vocabulary and general knowledge. This score was one factor in her placement in a special education class for children with learning disabilities in order to remediate deficits in all areas of language and reading. At the end of fourth grade, Cathy scored in the 20th percentile in reading. A year later, after the introduction of a structured phonics approach, Cathy's reading score rose to the 35th percentile.

As we worked, I struck a balance between the Orton Gillingham approach and the development of language and general knowledge that continued to be crucial if Cathy was to read with comprehension and be motivated to read at all. Language enrichment and meaningful reading permeated Cathy's special education classroom as well. Cathy's growing interest in increasing her vocabulary gave purpose to our work on phonics, which in turn accelerated Cathy's language development. The fact that reading and language reinforced one another in both classroom and resource room contributed to Cathy's growth in reading. Throughout, Cathy's motivated participation in a teaching-learning partnership was a key factor in her slow but consistent progress.

DOUGLAS

In the absence of language development during the first two years of life, profoundly deaf children remain at a "primitive and concrete level of communication and their cognitive development is unable to benefit from the expanded horizons to which language is the normal access" (Boothroyd 1988, 60–61). Such children are frequently "frustrated by their limited ability to externalize thoughts and wishes and by their lack of control over the social environment. They perceive themselves as being acted upon more than acting and may compensate by developing rigid and manipulative behaviours." The author cautions that children who do not have a viable language system by the time they are three or four years old are in "serious social and emotional jeopardy."

Douglas was such a child. Douglas was turning six when he entered the resource room. He had been diagnosed and fitted with hearing aids only a few months earlier. His delayed diagnosis had had a profound effect on his linguistic, social, and emotional development. Douglas entered school with a limited vocabulary of words and phrases. His speech, while generally intelligible to someone who knew what he was trying to say, was garbled and indistinct. Without hearing aids, Douglas' hearing loss was severe. With hearing aids, Douglas could hear and discriminate conversational speech at close range in a quiet setting. A highly structured phonics approach was instrumental in contributing to Douglas' growth in far-reaching and unanticipated ways.

A Budding Reader

From the beginning, Douglas had acquired and retained sight vocabulary with ease. He loved to read, and appeared to be a self-motivated learner. Walking down the hall in the spring of his kindergarten year, Douglas stopped short in front of a bulletin board, signaled me to wait, dropped down and extracted a small notebook from deep inside his sock, reached for a pencil stub in his pocket, jotted down whatever had caught his eye, and was ready to resume walking.

Douglas read solely on the strength of his sight vocabulary. He could make only minimal use of phonics clues in deciphering unfamiliar words. Lack of exposure to language had sharply curtailed Douglas' vocabulary, further hindering word recognition. Writing was limited to a small body of sight words.

A Discrepancy

What existed, then, was a discrepancy between Douglas' self-motivation and the reading skills needed if he was to succeed in independent learning. This gap was exacerbated by Douglas' need to control the learning situation. Handling Douglas left little energy for teaching or learning. His "wannas" and "dowannas" were nearly inflexible. Using a timer to divide the resource room session into four ten-minute segments helped depersonalize the situation.

Douglas progressed in reading during first grade, and ended the year reading beginning chapter books. The classroom teacher could not vouch for his comprehension, since Douglas was not responsive to being questioned about what he had read. He participated in group discussions only when coaxed, and avoided writing. The teacher's impression was that Douglas, while unquestionably intelligent, was "his own worst enemy."

A Learning Impasse

At the beginning of second grade, Douglas was as resistant to being part of an orderly line at bus time as he had been the previous year. Working together in the resource room felt a bit less tense. This lasted until I touched on areas and ways of working that provoked Douglas' resistance.

This presented a dilemma. On the one hand, Douglas—while mainstreamed in a regular second-grade class—had been hearing and developing language for only two years. The gaps in his learning and his inability to do all the work of the class were understandable and were, in fact, sympathetically understood by the classroom teacher. Douglas' frustrations and defenses in the face of this situation were also easy to understand.

On the other hand, Douglas rejected everything I offered that could help him past his learning impasses so that he could move ahead more easily and confidently. Axline (1964), reflecting on her work with emotionally disturbed children, comments that "when the initiative is left up to the individual, he will select the ground upon which he feels his greatest security" (p. 44). Reading together was Douglas' preferred activity. He tolerated discussing what we read as we went along. He was strongly opposed to approximating spelling, and rejected the auditory training and speech activities that could enable him to hear, articulate, and eventually write more accurately and independently. His resistance was unmitigated no matter how non-threatening I attempted to be.

Calling A Truce

As a power struggle began to reassert itself, I made the decision to make no demands that would create tension between us. I knew that Douglas could benefit from what I had to offer in order to become the learner he himself wanted to be. I also knew that locking horns with him would not move us closer to that goal, but would only sap my energy and deepen his resistance and frustration.

I was left with a single criterion for success: that resource room sessions be relaxed and pleasurable. This felt frustrating to me in view of Douglas' needs and my ability to help him meet them if only he would let me. But I held to this criterion because the alternative was exhausting and counterproductive. I also sensed that Douglas' own drive to learn could, if I gave it more scope, guide my attempts to help him.

A Fresh Start

Around that time, Douglas brought in a book of his own to read in the resource room. We read together, acting out parts of it to further comprehension, and excerpting essential vocabulary as we went along. "Halt, vile knave!" became one of Douglas' favorite phrases.

I then chose a book that had been a favorite of a number of beginning readers. *Brown Beauty* (Webster 1968) is the story of a horse who saves her farmer's life, proving that a horse can think for herself and can be a friend in a way that a tractor cannot. Douglas entered into the story reluctantly. But once he did, the story worked its own magic. It was the first undertaking that felt like a shared experience of which we were both part.

Next, Douglas selected *Bats in the Dark* (Kaufman 1972). He brought it to me with conviction and read it with fascination. It was my first clue as to Douglas' interest in the world of science and geography. Douglas allowed me to stop as frequently as needed to review earlier reading and clarify new vocabulary and concepts.

I made the next selection, and Douglas reacted defensively; but he was immediately drawn into *The Earth and the Sky* (Gallimard and Verdet 1989). The striking diagrams and transparencies, discussed in a minimum of clear and informative language, commanded his interest. Again Douglas allowed me to backtrack, clarify, and ascertain that the text made sense to him. Douglas brought his own questions, observations, and associations to this process.

Taking a Chance

I was heartened by our amicable and productive experiences with these books. I wondered whether Douglas would allow me to introduce some needed skills in conjunction with our reading together. I decided to try using the Orton Gillingham approach to acquaint Douglas with basic phonics concepts.

Something unexpected happened. Douglas' eyes lit up as I took out the first five cards and we began to chant, "*mitten* /m/, *fish* /f/, *apple* /a/. . . ." Here was a quick, snappy game he was willing to play. His interest extended to spelling the sounds from dictation, and to the oral and visual blending which, along with handwriting, are key elements of this method.

Douglas was not a beginning reader. He was a good reader in the making. What he needed was to consolidate the rudimentary phonics concepts he already had to some degree, and to build on that foundation. Because Douglas is hard of hearing, two additional factors were involved. He needed practice discriminating sounds auditorily. He also needed as much practice as he would tolerate in articulating sounds accurately.

A Ray of Light

It was crucial for Douglas that learning be free from the devastating failure that had characterized his life from the beginning. This meant safeguarding him from uncertainty and from the very possibility of error, both of which triggered willfulness out of proportion to the incident at hand. My acceptance of the gaps in Douglas' language and learning had not come close enough to being sensitive enough to this open wound.

Douglas' resistance made sense in view of the immeasurable powerlessness he must have felt every day of his life, in and out of school. This empathy became possible for me once I made the decision to remove all pressure from the resource room session, and could see Douglas begin to soften and to relate to me and to learning in a new way.

The sequential and cumulative nature of the Orton Gillingham approach was, itself, an advantage in this regard. The system provides its own direction, generates its own momentum, sets its own standards. This freed Douglas from the negative aspects of personal interaction. Whereas previously Douglas had stiffened up at attempts to help him correct his speech, he suddenly found auditory and speech work acceptable to the point that he began spontaneously to monitor his own articulation. A method that I had thought had little to offer children lacking in auditory discrimination and clarity of speech proved to be an avenue to these skills.

At the moment, we are continuing to build a repertory of sounds, with Douglas looking forward to this part of the resource room period.

ROBERT

The tentative success of a structured phonics approach with Douglas led me to try it with yet another child. Robert, a third grader, could read simple words and write some of them with varying degrees of accuracy. His speech was clear, reflecting his relatively mild hearing loss. Robert used phonics clues as best he could while writing. When reading, he was likely to respond to unfamiliar words with approximations or wild guesses. He backtracked to get information from the printed word only when he recognized that a phrase or sentence was not making sense. This happened only occasionally.

Robert's fluent language and intelligible speech gave the impression that his language was age appropriate. In fact, however, Robert's thinking was disorganized, often incoherent. His answers were seldom responsive to the questions. He could not pursue a thought for more than two sentences before his responses became scattered and unrelated. His comments during a conversation or discussion often seemed to come out of the blue, even when the topic was well within his knowledge and experience.

The following exchange took place at the beginning of fourth grade. I had written in our log about a situation that had occurred the day before: "I felt something tickling my arm. Then it flew away. It was a bee!"

Robert: You felt something ticking your arm?
Ms. S.:   Not ticking.
Robert: Ticking, walking away, tacking, tacky . . .
Ms. S.:   There's an 'l' in there; go back and look at the word.
Robert: . . . tickling.
Ms. S.:   What was it?
Robert: I don't know.
Ms. S.:   What does it say?
Robert: I felt . . . It was a bee.
Ms. S.:   So what happened?
Robert: I thought you said *you* flew away.

Pinpointing the Problem

When children's hearing proves unreliable, they stop listening. Robert's family did not support the consistent use of amplification. Children whose hearing fluctuates are at risk of developing auditory perception problems leading to inattention (Boothroyd 1988). This was a possible factor in Robert's lack of mental discipline. Beebe (1953) observed that if a child is asked to make up for what was missed in earlier years, the demands will prove too great and the child will not try to meet them.

While this has not been my experience in every case, it may have been true for Robert.

It took time to realize that what Robert needed was not instruction in reading, writing, or reasoning. He needed training in ruling out extraneous thoughts and irrelevant observations while attending to the task at hand. It occurred to me that the Orton Gillingham approach could provide a basis for this kind of work.

Robert was already comfortably familiar with consonant sounds. His knowledge of short vowels was tentative, but became more secure after a few weeks of auditory and visual discrimination exercises. It was spelling that exposed Robert's untrained auditory memory.

Spelling: A Route to Memory

Spelling from dictation reinforces children's knowledge of the sounds they are learning, and is a key component of the Orton Gillingham approach. Robert appeared to know short vowels, yet substituted one for another randomly when we first began our daily dictation that included sounds in isolation and three-letter words. Spelling together helped him sort out his confusion in a relatively short time.

Combining purposeful listening with active memory was new to Robert. The learning that resulted was different from any he had ever experienced before. For me, it was like hearing a child begin to use words that had previously been only in his or her passive vocabulary. It is as if the child has moved beyond the stage of learning, forgetting, and relearning to a solid and lasting knowledge of those words. In the same way, it felt as if Robert had come to know short vowels in a way that made me realize how uncertain his earlier "knowing" of them had been.

I continued to reinforce short vowels while introducing consonant blends. Again, Robert's writing showed the effects of diminished auditory discrimination due partly to hearing loss and partly to lack of concentration. We extended our work to the auditory discrimination of consonant blends through spelling dictation.

Beyond Penmanship

In the Orton Gillingham approach, spelling goes hand in hand with penmanship. The kinesthetic aspect of letter formation reinforces sound-symbol associations, which are difficult for dyslexic children to acquire. I suspected that, for Robert, focusing on handwriting could serve an additional purpose.

Robert's writing could be reasonably neat and legible. But there was little regard for size and placement of letters or method of letter formation. I believed that strict attention to a standardized system of forming letters could help build the concentration Robert so sorely needed.

Going back to primary paper enabled Robert to see more clearly the relationship of letters to lines and spaces. He followed along as I talked him through the correct starting point, ending point, and direction of pencil strokes for each letter. After several weeks of dictation, Robert had begun to form letters with care and accuracy, independently, and with a sense of confidence.

I wonder whether this was the first time in his life that Robert ever felt secure in knowing what he was doing. It is my hope that pursuing this highly structured approach to reading and writing will help develop in him the internal organization that could lead to success in other areas of learning.

SUMMING UP

As a teacher of children whose vocabulary, syntax, articulation, and comprehension are affected by hearing loss, I have strongly favored a language-centered approach to reading. My initial experience with a highly structured phonics method has given me information and know-how that I now realize had been missing from my understanding as a teacher of reading. This way of working has offered security and mastery to the very children I had avoided burdening with too pointed a phonics approach.

Chall (1967, 307) emphasizes that "the evidence *does not endorse any one code-emphasis method over another.*" An Orton Gillingham course, offered at a convenient time, led me to this particular form of instruction.

The Orton Gillingham approach, among others, contains elements that have characterized other successful teaching-learning endeavors.

- Its structure gives shape to a range of skills that some children are unable to deduce without direct teaching.
- The carefully paced progression provides children with a sense of security and mastery.

- Concepts are touched on, rather than dwelt on, again and again in a variety of contexts.
- Progress is systematic and tangible.

REFLECTIONS

My experience with the Orton Gillingham approach suggests that there is reason to give those children whose hearing allows for it, the benefit of phonics instruction. Chall (1967) challenged the belief that a child's interest in reading particular stories is the key to his or her desire to develop reading skills. The children whom she observed were "as excited and keenly interested in words, sounds, spellings, and rules as they were in stories" (p. 270). Chall noted that children lost interest in words beyond their comprehension, but became eagerly involved when interesting and familiar words were used as the basis for practicing reading skills. This has been my experience as well.

Reading speed is a factor in comprehension. Anderson et al. (1985) have determined that third graders read aloud at an average rate of 100 words per minute; a rate of 50 to 72 words per minute is "so slow as to interfere with comprehension even of easy material" (p. 13). Attending to the mechanics of written material is "unlikely to leave much . . . capacity free for developing new comprehension abilities." Adding even rudimentary phonics knowledge to a core of sight words has resulted in significant gains in reading speed and fluency for several children.

In any discipline, the process of developing and refining skills leading to mastery is not merely a means to an end, but a source of pleasure and satisfaction in its own right. This is as true for young readers as for learners of all ages and stages, in all fields of endeavor.

"Robert loves syllable division so much that he wants to do it even if he doesn't need to," I commented to Cathy with amusement. "I don't blame him," she responded instantly. Robert's engagement with this basic skill and Cathy's heartfelt response reveal their excitement in learning to read, as well as their appreciation of the kind of teaching that is making it possible.

In a short time, I have seen the promise of a multisensory approach to phonics for children who do not come to decoding easily because of problems that include, but are not limited to, learning disabilities. Language remains the most basic educational need of children who are deaf and hard of hearing. Adding a structured phonics approach to my repertoire of teaching skills has given me the knowledge and methodology I need to increase the children's level of comfort with reading, making integrated language learning more accessible to them.

For a child who is shut off from reading and learning by a serious inability to decode, multisensory phonics instruction is a gift. This was impressed upon me by Cathy.

After four months of phonics work, Cathy arrived at school in a state of excitement. She could hardly contain herself. "I'm so proud of myself, I can't believe it!" she announced. She repeated this over and over on our way to the resource room. Once inside, she shared with me that she had read half a biography of Amelia Earhart and written half a book report entirely on her own. "My mother couldn't believe that I wrote it by myself," she wrote in the log. "But of cors I didn't coppy from the book. I never coppy from the book."

Cathy reminded me of an experience I had completely forgotten. Two years earlier, when she was in third grade and could barely read, we had made our way through a different biography of Amelia Earhart to fulfill a Women's History Month assignment. I did the reading, and we discussed it together.

Soon after that, we spent a number of sessions reading and discussing *Living in Prehistoric Times* (Chisholm 1982). I recall asking Cathy what Amelia Earhart might have accomplished if she had lived in those days and had the same qualities that enabled her to become an airplane pilot. Cathy thought about it, then responded that she might have been the first woman to tame a wild dog. I remember being surprised and impressed by her answer.

Cathy showed me her report and described Amelia Earhart's life. Her pride was justified. She was reading and writing on a level she had never come close to before, and she was aware of it.

On our way back to class, Cathy couldn't help letting me know once again how proud she was feeling. I told her that she deserved to feel proud of herself, partly because of the quality of her work, and partly because she had kept on trying all those years when learning had been hard for her. Now, at last, she was beginning to see the results of her perseverance. Cathy was silent for a moment, then said softly, "I thought I would always be a nobody. . . ." As we walked, she raised her head and proclaimed: " . . . and now I want to be a doctor and a teacher and an artist and a writer!"

With these words, a child who only a short time before had been drowning in a sea of letters she could not decipher, paid moving tribute to a method that had brought her her first experience of reading, pride, and hope.

Chapter 19

Untangling the Web

Multifaceted problems rooted in a variety of sources are baffling by their very nature. They require educational and psychological detective work to unravel. I have found that clearing up even a small part of any problem area allows others to emerge more clearly. Gradually, some difficulties are reduced or eliminated, while others come more clearly into focus and can be addressed in turn.

DOMINIQUE

Dominique, for whom "having a conversation" had been the first step in learning to focus her attention on the task at hand, entered the resource room program in kindergarten. I met her during registration. Dominique had a mild-to-moderate hearing loss that was substantially corrected by hearing aids. My impression that she was intellectually slow soon gave way to uncertainty.

While her mother was filling out record cards, I let Dominique know that she would need to bring a bookbag, a notebook, and her lunch to school the next day. I then asked her to tell me what she needed to bring. There was a long silence. Something made me hold back and resist the temptation to put the words in her mouth.

Seconds went by, then: ". . . a bookbag"; ". . . a notebook"; and finally, ". . . my lunch." The lag between Dominique's hearing my question, making sense out of it, and formulating a response suggested a breakdown in a process that normally takes place so smoothly that we are not conscious of the steps involved. By managing to respond appropriately, Dominique had given the first hint of the "checkerboard of weaknesses and strengths" (Murphy 1982) that characterized this globally disabled child and her learning processes.

Strengths and Needs

Early on, Dominique revealed specific strengths that stood out in comparison with her more obvious disabilities. She tossed off reciting the alphabet, days of the week, and months of the year. She counted easily from 1 to 100. Rote memory was and would remain her greatest asset. Although Dominique volunteered little in the way of spontaneous communication, she usually responded to direct questioning. Her answers revealed that she was informed about her home and family life, and showed some social awareness.

In contrast, basic motor skills were far less developed. Thus, Dominique's first lesson at school was descending stairs using alternate feet. Several years later, on an educational evaluation, Dominique scored 1 out of 10 in alternate-foot hopping. She could hop on her right foot and on her left, but couldn't figure out how to make the switch.

This extreme deficit in the fundamental area of body awareness was accompanied by deficits of equal magnitude in every area of learning. One of these was an absence of number orientation so profound that, years later, one-to-one correspondence still had no meaning for her.

Dominique's ability to perceive the world around her was impaired in two major areas. The first was visual and spatial. She could not copy simple geometric shapes. The second was auditory. In spite of having a good deal of hearing, Dominique had extreme difficulty focusing her attention in a situation that involved listening. At such times, her gaze would wander and her body begin to move until she had twisted herself off the chair and onto the floor. This was not a behavior problem, but a literal representation in body language of how far her mind had strayed.

Dominique seemed barely in touch with teacher-directed classroom activities. Yet weeks after Columbus Day had passed, she was overheard by her mother picking up her toy telephone, dialing Queen Isabella, and confronting her: "Hello, Queen

Isabella? Where's the money for those ships you were going to send me?" The fact that she had taken in that information, retained it, and made it her own was a surprising and amusing indication of Dominique's capacity for learning.

A Need for Focus

Throughout kindergarten, first grade, and into second we worked in a variety of areas. First steps in reading, while slow in coming, were tentatively encouraging and inspired confidence in both of us. Math, because of its spatial nature, yielded no such satisfaction. Always, Dominique's need to learn to mobilize her attention was uppermost.

In this connection, two threads ran through the first several years of resource room work. The first of these was my reading stories aloud sentence by sentence, and having Dominique repeat each sentence word for word. Slowly, Dominique's ability to attend to the speaker improved and her auditory memory became stronger. Eventually it became easy for her to give back several lengthy sentences at a time. The second ongoing activity was learning to have a simple conversation. This process is described in Chapter 2.

During these activities, it was constantly necessary to focus and refocus Dominique's attention on the person speaking. In the two-and-one-half years that we kept coming back to these two activities, I felt that I was groping in the dark. There was little feedback to confirm that what I was doing was actually of value.

One day, as Dominique and I were working together, I began to feel frustrated and discouraged that she was fingering the ribbon of her dress. Suddenly I realized that her body was in the chair, her eyes and ears were in good contact with what we were working on, and that she was doing nothing more serious than fidgeting with her bow. At that moment it became clear for the first time that our work thus far had contributed to laying the groundwork for a new quality of attention which, in turn, would perhaps make other kinds of learning possible.

JERRY

Being unable to learn and wanting not to are as different as night and day. Children who have something invested in not learning may ward off the most earnest attempts to help them succeed. While doing well in school may be their deepest wish, it remains hidden and unattainable as long as some inner obstacle pushes it beyond reach.

Like Dominique, Jerry was remarkable because of his extraordinary difficulty in focusing his attention. But what appeared to be a similar problem gradually revealed itself as being very different.

Before transferring to the resource room program, Jerry had completed kindergarten and half of first grade in his neighborhood school. English was not Jerry's home language. He seemed to understand basic English, but spoke little. Jerry had a mild to moderate hearing loss. With hearing aids, his ability to understand what people were saying was good, as long as background noise was not overwhelming. In the classroom, wearing an FM unit minimized this problem.

A Cause for Concern

Because of his limited command of English, Jerry was placed in kindergarten as the setting most conducive to developing language. Long past the initial stages of acquiring English, he continued to communicate only minimally. In June of second grade, it occurred to me that it would be revealing to keep a record of Jerry's spontaneous utterances. While I regretted not having thought of this earlier, I could almost compile such a list using my imagination. Entries would be sparse and might have included the following: "Drink water? Leave? Take a book? Jason's absent?"

What struck me as worth understanding more deeply was not only how little Jerry volunteered in the way of verbal communication, but even more, the nature of what he did say.

A Confusing Picture

It was striking that Jerry tended to express himself tersely, using as few words as possible to get his message across. This did not reflect his grasp of English, since he was also capable of letting me know: "Yesterday you told me that today you were going to give me a surprise." But full-length sentences were rare, and monosyllabic communications predominated.

The question form was characteristic of Jerry. "What shall we start with today?" I asked. "Maybe . . . word box?" he might reply hesitantly. "How much are 1 + 1, Jerry?" I asked him. "Maybe . . . 2?" he ventured. Through tentative answers such as these, Jerry seemed to convey a need to ensure approval. Other questions were aimed at securing immediate wants. What seemed to be lacking were questions and observations indicating a broader interest and awareness, such as are shown by even much younger children as they begin to experience other people and the world around them. There were exceptions. Jerry mentioned with pleasure a family outing to the beach, and details of his brother's First Communion. There were perhaps four such moments of sharing while he was in second grade.

In the Classroom

Several times Jerry also spoke up unexpectedly when other children in the class were being quietly remonstrated. Suddenly he revealed his alertness to what was going on, as well as a lively and insistent interest in the stringency of the punishment. These incidents were doubly surprising: partly because his voice was so seldom heard; and partly because they indicated an awareness of his school world that was otherwise barely in evidence.

Jerry's connectedness with classroom life and learning was limited by a startling lack of purposeful focusing. His second-grade teacher estimated that he brought his attention to the activity at hand no more than a few minutes each day. Other than that, he came close to being a non-participant in the classroom in spite of continuous attempts to involve him in a wide variety of small-group, large-group, and individual activities. Observers in and out of the classroom were struck by the extent of Jerry's inattention, as well as by his lack of eye contact.

In the Resource Room

Resource room work during Jerry's first several years of school felt like a trail of false starts in various areas using a variety of approaches. Perhaps because he revealed himself so little, I did not succeed in taking my cue from Jerry, in picking up on what was close to his heart and using his own interests as taking-off points for learning. At the same time, while Jerry appeared outwardly compliant, the impetus for continuing with activities initiated by me came mainly from me. It was as if nothing in Jerry took over to breathe life into them and make them his own. As a result, I began and dropped activity after activity.

Two activities came closest to capturing and maintaining Jerry's interest. The first was keeping a shoebox of sight vocabulary words that he reviewed, checked off daily, and retired after three checks. The second was developing vocabulary through pictures following the same system. Jerry kept a tally of these by coloring in the number of words learned each day on a hundred-square.

We worked on the sight words during the first half or three-quarters of the year. Jerry was business-like in taking out, reading through, and checking his words. I grasped at picture vocabulary toward the end of the year on the basis of its success with another child. Again, Jerry would take the initiative in spreading out his pictures on the table and naming them each day. By reviewing his words quite regularly in the evenings, he mastered one hundred words in a relatively short time.

Both of these activities seemed productive and satisfying. Yet the sight vocabulary lost its momentum and petered out. The picture vocabulary, even though the immediate goal of one hundred words was achieved, also left me feeling at a loss. It was as if each of them lost the quality of freshness that would have encouraged me to continue. Neither gave rise to any insight as to how to proceed from there. In not generating their own growth, they lost their early promise and became static.

I believe that the two vocabulary projects succeeded as well as they did for two reasons: once the teacher's hand was removed, the remaining structure was unchanging and impersonal; and no language or thinking skills beyond rote memory were demanded. In a way, the very qualities that made these activities accessible and acceptable to Jerry were ultimately limiting and growth-defeating.

Looking Deeper

Jerry's difficulties were multifaceted. Hearing loss and having English as a second language were contributing factors. But they played only a part in this eight-and-one-half-year-old boy's scoring in the four-year-old range on an English evaluation of vocabulary and sentence structure. In his home language, Jerry could not achieve the minimum score required for testing to proceed. Language impairment, an aspect of learning disability that interferes with the natural development of language, was a possibility. Yet the same child found the words to express himself as fully as needed in both languages when something of pressing personal interest was at stake. This discrepancy made it seem likely that emotional factors were affecting the extent and form of Jerry's communication, his ability to focus, and his learning.

The youngest of three sons, Jerry had been deeply affected at age two by the birth of his sister. The caring attention he received was not sufficient to reassure him of his niche in the family and of his place in his parent's affection. This was borne out by glimpses of well-contained but potentially explosive anger. Jerry gave voice to his resentment in a card to a classmate whose grandfather had died. His message was: "I hope your mother dies." What felt like a committed avoidance of focusing and communication seemed to be symbolic of this inner stance toward adults in authority. Jerry was much freer in his interactions with children.

The emotional factors that seemed to hold the key to understanding and reaching Jerry were beyond my competence to deal with as a teacher. This realization did not solve the impasse. But it freed me of the burden of responsibility for finding the solution on my own, and led to Jerry's participation in a family-oriented mental health program. It was also helpful to realize that Jerry's and my work together, while it felt lacking in direction, might contribute to future growth. Perhaps first steps toward being able to learn freely were taking place, even then, in ways that could not yet be observed and measured. Perhaps one day it would become possible to see how growth and learning had their roots in this difficult stage.

JIMMY

Jimmy's hearing loss was identified at age two-and-one-half. By the time he entered kindergarten and the resource room program, he had two years of speech and language therapy and several years of nursery school behind him.

Jimmy had a profound hearing loss with some usable hearing. He generally understood what was said to him as long as the language was kept simple and was clearly connected to what was going on at the moment. He himself shyly volunteered a few words here and there, usually indistinctly and in a low voice. Slowly, Jimmy began to use whole sentences to relate an experience or express his reaction to a story. Typical of young

deaf children, his sentences consisted of key words strung together. A visit to relatives became "Jimmy-Mommy-train
Grandma house."

A Child in Need

After discovering that Jimmy had some good rudimentary
language, something began to puzzle me. I noticed that he could
barely answer specific questions based on the same conversation
that had given rise to a spontaneous outpouring of language
only a moment earlier. In addition, his vocabulary was far more
limited than might be expected, even of a deaf child who had
had several years of work in language development.

Jimmy had attended a neighborhood nursery school for two
years before entering kindergarten. Yet complying with class routines seemed to be something entirely new and foreign to him.
Difficulty in following verbal directions and attending to group
lessons was understandable in view of his hearing loss. But hearing loss did not fully account for his defiant refusal to comply in
self-explanatory situations or when directions were made clear
and concrete. It did not account for his pouting and withdrawal
when expected to take turns. Neither did it explain his sometimes overt, often furtive striking out at other children without
apparent provocation (this alongside of demonstrations of genuine sweetness and concern). Seemingly benign pictures and
events aroused gleeful recitals of real and imaginary violence.

In the Resource Room

Much of this could be observed in the resource room as
well. It felt as if there must be some missing clue without which
we were at a loss to understand the variety and extent of the interpersonal difficulties and difficulty in sustaining attention that
Jimmy revealed in school.

In the course of searching for a language-expanding activity that would put us on the right track, I reached for *I Spy*
(Ogle 1970). This was a beginning word book with two life-like
drawings of common objects per page. I opened the book to the
first page and asked Jimmy to name each picture. As with Jerry,
I drew unfamiliar items on cards that he took home in an envelope to learn that evening. From then on, Jimmy began each day
by spreading out all his pictures on the table and identifying as
many as he could. As he named a picture, I gave it a check in

the corner. Pictures with three checks were considered learned and were taken home for good.

I delayed addressing Jimmy's second area of need—his difficulty answering specific questions—until our work with vocabulary had been securely established.

Signs of Change

As the weeks went by, I began to notice some changes in Jimmy. His behavior became organized and purposeful, qualities that had been conspicuously lacking. He would stride across the room to the table and be seated expectantly by the time I had covered the distance from the door to the far side of the room. He attended patiently as Dominique went through her words, and calmly and efficiently spread out his own when his turn came.

With his mother's help, Jimmy was regular in working on his words and returning them to school every morning. As drawing, learning, and checking became an established pattern, negative interpersonal behavior decreased and, eventually, completely ceased. Understandably, behaviors that diminished in the controlled setting of the resource room persisted in the much more stimulating and demanding classroom situation.

Whenever I thought of adding variety to our daily session, something cautioned me against it. Because our work together felt easy and relaxed and I was reluctant to risk going back to a frustrating situation, I continued along from one day to the next without deviating from this pattern.

Clarifying the Picture

Jimmy lived with his parents and older brother in a one-room apartment. I had hints of the noisiness and disorganization that were part of this difficult situation. I was aware that his mother's caring concern, compounded by stress, was mixed with extreme overprotectiveness. In time, these impressions were confirmed by the psychologist who was working with the troubled older brother and with the family as a whole. The psychologist also shared relevant information regarding family dynamics.

This was the enlightening "missing link." It was then that some of what I had sensed but not fully understood became clear. I realized that the vocabulary gained from our work, while beneficial to Jimmy, was secondary to the value of the fixed routine itself. Chaos was so pervasive and so deeply rooted in his existence that nothing less than week after week of utter simplicity and predictability could have given him the experience of stability needed for his own inner sense of structure to emerge. This, in turn, gave rise to a deserved sense of accomplishment.

The vocabulary experiment went on unchanged for six months. It enriched Jimmy's vocabulary by about two hundred words. Yet the dramatic altering of behavior and attitude took place in the first two months. Part of the original puzzle remained: why Jimmy, with his residual hearing, consistent amplification, and early intervention, did not make greater progress in the areas of speech and language.

Most deaf and hard-of-hearing children are socially, emotionally, and intellectually intact. Others may manifest serious difficulties in more than one area. Distinguishing between primary and secondary problems, and coming to understand their interrelationship, is seldom a quick or an easy task. Imposing structure of one kind or another has helped me find my way in such situations.

Chapter 20

When Resource Room is Not Enough

The gap between young deaf and hard-of-hearing resource room children and their hearing classmates is often tremendous. Children with hearing impairments may lack basic vocabulary and conversational skills. They may be unable to count or recite the alphabet. They may be inexperienced in following a story, and have a minimum of comprehension. Addressing these areas in a gradual and consistent way can create a foundation that leads to successful mainstreaming.

Occasionally, a child's deficits are too great, and his or her rate of learning too slow, for mainstreaming to be beneficial. It then becomes the resource room teacher's responsibility to arrive at the clearest possible understanding of the child's abilities in order to determine the setting that will meet his or her needs most effectively.

A number of children who began in regular classrooms with resource room support have moved on to more appropriate placements. Nancy is such a child.

NANCY

As babies grow, a succession of needs begins to assert itself. Corresponding skills normally develop to meet these needs. For example, toddlers have an urgent need to make their wishes known. They accomplish this with the help of their growing vocabulary. Boothroyd (1988) calls this correspondence "developmental synchrony."

In contrast, developmental asynchrony occurs when skills are not available to meet particular needs. Children who lack the language needed to interact with people may achieve their desires by tantrums and other manipulative behavior. With children who are deaf and hard of hearing, early language development acts to preserve developmental synchrony, thereby fostering social development.

Nancy, who was enrolled in the resource room program at the beginning of the school year, displayed evidence of developmental asynchrony. About to turn six, she had just been fitted with hearing aids for a severe hearing loss. Without them, she heard little and had developed no language.

Several hours in a first grade class revealed antisocial behavior, along with a general inability to understand and follow fundamental classroom procedures. Nancy's family agreed to a kindergarten placement in order to provide her with the kinds of language and social experiences she needed.

Getting Started

In the resource room, our first task was to develop basic vocabulary. Nancy, now wearing hearing aids, had begun to pick up situationally related language. When I held her hand against her will because she tended to run away, she swiftly let me know that "My Mommy gonna beat your. . . ." At the same time, Nancy was unable to identify such items as table, chair, boy, girl, dog, or cat in a picture dictionary.

We began going through the dictionary systematically, and drawing picture cards of each item that Nancy could not name. These picture cards, reviewed and reinforced daily in school and at home, introduced Nancy to the names of familiar objects.

Expanding Language

The pictures also provided opportunities to move beyond labeling. "Pick up the key," I said one morning, glancing at the large key that I had drawn and Nancy had cut out. "Knock on the door," I demonstrated. Nancy raced over to the classroom door and knocked delightedly. "Nobody's home!" I reported. Nancy shrugged her shoulders dramatically, looking appropriately forlorn. "Where's the key?" I continued. "Turn the key. . . . Open the door. . . . You opened the door! My turn." We reenacted the scene, Nancy directing me to knock, take the key out of my pocket, turn it, and open the door.

Nancy could not get enough of this kind of play. I supplied the language, and she happily mimicked it back to me. In spite of a lifetime of disuse, Nancy's auditory memory was unimpaired. A growing number of words and phrases took on meaning for her.

Aiming Higher

Gradually Nancy's vocabulary grew to encompass a variety of colors, toys, animals, foods, and pieces of furniture. I was excited by the prospect of using these familiar words as the basis for a higher level of language work. One day I drew a cow, then an elephant in her notebook. On the opposite page I drew an apple and a banana. I attempted to elicit from Nancy the names of other animals, other foods to add to these groups, but she was unable to bring her word knowledge to bear on this task.

On a separate card I drew a cat and placed it questioningly first in one group, then in the other. This did not clarify the concept of "belonging" for Nancy in this context. Her ability to categorize was evident from her interaction with her surroundings. She was as clear about the appropriate use of objects in her environment as any child her age. Yet Nancy had begun to acquire language only six months earlier. Despite her obvious intelligence and rapid rate of vocabulary growth, she did not yet have a way of using words to think about concepts that she would have been likely to grasp in nonverbal situations.

The Next Step

Story reading was also affected by Nancy's language limitations. Reading together had not become another avenue to language development. Early picture books, books with repetitive refrains—all were beyond Nancy's ability to follow and enjoy. No book was simple enough for this six-year-old with the language and behavior of a toddler until I found *Mommy, Where Are You?* (Ziefert 1988). On each page, Little Hippo calls to his mother. A flap lifts up and there, behind the door, gate, or shower curtain is Mommy Hippo.

Nancy's involvement in the story was immediate and complete. She worried along with Baby Hippo, and was relieved and delighted as we turned back the flaps and exclaimed, "There she is!" We read the story every day for weeks. Nancy's reactions made it clear that here was finally a book that satisfied her linguistic and emotional needs.

Having been reassigned from first grade to kindergarten, Nancy could not be held over again. By the end of the year, she had the beginnings of a working vocabulary, but was far from ready to experience success in a regular first grade class. In the spring of her kindergarten year, Nancy was transferred to a self-contained class for deaf and hard-of-hearing children. This setting offered the opportunity she needed to continue her language development and move on from there.

JOSHUA

Joshua, with his difficulty remembering words and mastering the alphabet, had just turned seven when he entered the resource room program. His mild to moderate hearing loss had been recently diagnosed. His brand-new hearing aids were still at home, as yet unworn.

Joshua was to repeat first grade, since he had learned little in his first-grade class the previous year. His mother advised me that I would need patience with him as a learner. I tried picturing what is must be like for a little boy with an unidentified hearing loss to sit passively in school, day after day, while the work of the class went on around him.

First Impressions

My first impression of Joshua was that he had a fair amount of conversational language. At the end of the first day of school he queried, "The bus come—Mommy home?" I reassured him that the bus would take him home and Mommy would be waiting for him. This seemed to satisfy him.

Our school corridors have double doors. I sometimes remind the children to use the door on the right so as not to get hit by children bursting through the other door from the opposite side. During the early days of school, I overheard Joshua cautioning the other children, "You have to use this door; otherwise you might get hit." While this was something Joshua had heard me say, he remembered it accurately and used it appropriately. This, and similar language, had been acquired without the benefit of hearing aids, which Joshua had just begun to wear. It seemed to bode well for his ability to pick up language and make it his own.

Warning Signals

Joshua actively observed and made sense of his surroundings. He demonstrated a grasp of how the world works. At the same time, it was becoming apparent that he lacked the vocabulary to put this "inner language" into words. When shown a picture of a stamped envelope, Joshua explained: "You put the thing on the thing, then you put it in the mailbox, then you open the thing with a key and you take out a video."

Joshua could follow simple directions and answer simple questions. His comprehension was held back by his severely limited word knowledge. He could not identify the most common of objects. He could answer the question "What color?" yet could not differentiate between "What color?" and "What shape?" even after several weeks of exposure to this language concept.

Joshua's language was often imprecise: "If you put them like that" (referring to the placement of picture cards in the envelope), "then we can't put the notebook" (close the notebook). In describing a picture of a boy eating an ice cream cone, Joshua explained, "He's licking it so it could fall off." Asked to name what two children in pajamas were wearing, Joshua's response was, "Then you sleep with bed."

Joshua had extraordinary difficulty retaining new vocabulary, even when exposed to a word for days at a time in a variety of contexts. He could sometimes supply information about words he was unable to name: "When somebody do that, that means you have to line up" (bell); I have one like that" (drum). At times, a description gave him the prompting he needed to come up with a word: "When you paint, you put on a . . . (smock)." At other times, memory failed him: "When it's hot, you turn on the . . . ('feather' for 'fan')." Yet once "feather" was clarified, the word was no more available to him than "fan" had been.

At times it was possible to see that Joshua's responses made sense if only he could fill in what he was leaving out. At other times it was not possible to follow his thought process. While picking up a flannel-board cutout of a bed, Joshua volunteered, "I know what this is—a pumpkin. Sometimes they look like a bed" (pointing to the rectangular empty space of the headboard).

Further Difficulties

For Joshua, reading was not a viable route to language development at this point. His mother had been correct in observing that it would take patience to teach him his "abc's." In September, Joshua could recite the alphabet but was able to identify only half the letters. By January, he could point out and name most of the letters. By mid-year, left-to-right progression had become established. On the other hand, one-to-one correspondence between written and spoken words was not yet consistent. At times, Joshua moved his finger along while retelling "I - like - Mommy." At other times, he would go off into a long narrative while pointing to a single word.

Joshua recognized his name in print. With the possible exception of "Mommy," "no," "go," and "I," he had no other sight vocabulary. Joshua was aware that initial consonants provide a clue to word meaning, but could not identify the sounds of particular consonants. When reviewing a picture of mittens, he volunteered: "*m* begins with the letter 'mitten.'" Another day he circled the first letter of *truck*, explaining that *m* begins with the letter 'truck.'"

A Necessary Placement

Joshua's communication delay appeared to be related to difficulties in perception and memory. This condition, when severe, has been described as "childhood aphasia." Joshua did not respond to the kinds of activities through which deaf and hard-of-hearing children begin to develop language. His hearing loss was secondary to his communication disorder. The severity of the delays in Joshua's language, as well as in auditory and visual perception and memory, necessitated placement in a small class whose primary focus was to train children in the acquisition and use of language.

EMILY

Over the years, Emily demonstrated a variety of difficulties in addition to those typically associated with her mild-to-moderate hearing loss. It was necessary to focus and refocus her attention even in the one-to-one resource room setting. By the middle of second grade, Emily had begun to sustain attention to reading, listening, and thinking activities for several minutes at a time. At those times, her vagueness was replaced by lively and alert participation. By fourth grade, Emily was in good contact with resource room tasks part of the time, although fidgeting and distractibility persisted. Emily's increased ability to focus in the resource room setting did not extend to the classroom, where she continued to have difficulty paying attention.

A Range of Disabilities

As early as kindergarten, Emily showed a compelling interest in learning to read. She acquired sight vocabulary easily. Consonant recognition enabled her to decode semifamiliar words with the help of context clues. Because of her weak auditory memory, Emily had real difficulty retaining the sounds of short vowels. Her own misarticulations ("pit" for *put*, "opple" for *apple*) contributed to the problem. These mispronunciations were idiosyncratic and not those typically associated with hearing impairment.

Emily's visual memory was also weak. By age nine, she had not acquired the standard spellings of words that come easily to many younger children through repeated exposure.

Emily could count by rote and had some math vocabulary. In second grade, however, she still lacked such basic concepts as "Which is more, 2 or 9?" Two years later, she had not yet developed number constancy. For example, having found that the blue and the white Cuisinaire rods were equal in length to the orange rod, Emily could not reverse the process and conceptualize what to put with the white rod to match the orange. This developmental stage is usually achieved by age six or seven.

Signs of Language Impairment

Emily's language contained some errors related to hearing loss, while others seemed characteristic of language impairment. These included misuse of pronouns ("The boy was running; she fell down") and misuse of prepositions ("The book fell out the table"). When such errors were brought to Emily's attention, she could sometimes correct herself. Similarly, when her own sentences were modeled back to her, she was sometimes able to make corrections and completions (from "The first little pig went on the second little pig" to "The first little pig went to the house of the second little pig").

Emily had difficulty making her answers responsive to questions. By the end of second grade she had improved in this area, though not yet consistently. "What did the children have for supper?" I asked as we read *The Boxcar Children* (Warner

1989) together. "They was going to have supper after dinner," Emily responded.

Emily's language revealed errors in syntax. She correctly identified categories, but within a given category used specific words interchangeably. For example, when asked how a child might feel if her best friend moved away, she responded "happy." During our reading of *The Boxcar Children*, Henry was busy making a broom. When asked what Henry was making with the branches, Emily answered, "Like you sweep the vacuum."

In time, Emily became better able to elaborate on what she had read or experienced. Her short-term memory was stronger than her long-term memory. She often had little or no recall of what she had read or discussed a day or two earlier, even with the help of leading questions or relating what had gone on up to that point.

While Emily was gaining in her ability to relate a sequence of events, she had difficulty distinguishing relevant from less relevant information and connecting her sentences in a way that made sense: "Once there were three little pigs. A man came walking by. The first one he did it with sticks."

Moving On

Emily's accomplishments in a variety of areas testified to her ability as a learner. But even with resource room support, her progress in a regular classroom did not reflect her potential. At the beginning of fourth grade, Emily joined a small class for hearing children with learning disabilities.

Chapter 21

Fitting It All In

The 45-minute resource room period is both generous and frustrating. Of all mainstreamed children with special needs, only hearing-impaired students have the luxury of daily individual or small-group remedial instruction. Yet even this does not begin to meet the needs of many deaf and hard-of-hearing children.

Hearing-related deficits and class curriculum provide the field from which resource room instruction is drawn. But even targeting specific areas leaves more than can be addressed in a session or series of sessions.

On the one hand, it is essential to make intense and efficient use of time. On the other hand, it takes "a lot of slow" for learning to take place and be absorbed and integrated.

How can we achieve a balance between the efficiency of a clinical session and the leisure essential to growth and learning? How can we move children along as quickly as possible, while creating a relaxed and unpressured atmosphere in which we seem to have all the time in the world?

This paradox is a major challenge of resource room teaching.

TAKING STOCK

Addressing several areas one after the other is a logical use of resource room time. This format provides variety and contrast, which help keep sessions lively and dynamic.

At times, keeping a number of activities going at once deteriorates into an unsuccessful juggling act. This often signals a mismatch between the work of the moment and the child's current level. It is also an inevitable consequence of trying to cover too much. I have found boredom and frustration on my part to be valuable indicators of the need to reassess the scope and pace of resource room work.

Examining the child's needs and behaviors, my own teaching agenda, and the interplay between the two may lead to adjusting ways of working and/or my expectations. This sometimes entails making the difficult decision to sacrifice some areas in order to work more comfortably on others.

The following descriptions of resource room sessions depict a range of activities and the thinking behind them.

THREE TYPICAL RESOURCE ROOM SESSIONS

Cathy

In fifth grade, Cathy was just beginning to read and write with a degree of fluency and competence. A multisensory phonics approach was succeeding where other attempts had failed. Knowing that Cathy's family would be moving to another part of the country, I wished to give her as many decoding tools as I could in the few remaining months of school. Yet language and background information vied for attention with the mechanics of reading. All three were essential to Cathy's growth as a learner and as a person.

Vocabulary was not a tedious exercise as far as Cathy was concerned. Her word cards were out of her notebook and in front of her by the time I had taken off my coat and arrived at the table. Her interest in the contents of each card was palpable. Cathy read some words easily and worked her way through others. One word or phrase led to a discussion that enriched her understanding. Another evoked a moment of shared humor. It seemed clear that Cathy felt quietly empowered by her expanding knowledge and by her growing supply of words with which to express it.

For several days, we had been moving from vocabulary to consolidating familiar phonics concepts and introducing new ones. Today, though, I noticed that most of Cathy's vocabulary cards had three checks and were ready to be "retired," leaving only a few words in her envelope. Word attack skills are of dubious value without corresponding growth in language and general knowledge. So, for the moment, I postponed further work on decoding in favor of some "real" reading.

Cathy perused two newspaper articles. She passed up the story of a football star with one arm in favor of an article that captured her interest in several respects. Two signing deaf teachers from a neighboring school for the deaf had been summoned by police to a nearby rooftop. Their two-hour dialogue saved the life of a despondent deaf man about to commit suicide. Cathy and I began to read. The article provoked discussion, and was a source of new vocabulary. Some words yielded to Cathy's prowess as a reader with budding word attack skills. With others, help was needed. All were meaningful to her.

Our time was over. Cathy packed up her vocabulary cards, which her mother would hear that evening. We had become so absorbed in reading that I had forgotten to leave time for each of us to write in our group log. As we walked back to class, Cathy yawned. She explained that she had been up during the night comforting her little brother, who had awakened with a nightmare. Cathy's depiction of her brother's fear and her response as a big sister were vivid and sympathetic. I asked her to remember her words and write that story for the log.

Joshua

In spite of his having only a mild to moderate hearing loss, Joshua's extreme difficulty retaining words persisted throughout his second year of first grade. A previous teacher had noted that Joshua could recite the alphabet but identify only half the letters. While this was true, it felt more important to use our time to develop as much of a language foundation as possible. The alphabet could wait.

In the early spring, Joshua himself gravitated toward a wooden alphabet puzzle I had recently acquired. He began session after session by taking "his" puzzle and challenging himself to sequence the letters once, twice, and sometimes three times in a row. Joshua's independence, persistence, and the intensity of his involvement indicated that this task answered needs in several areas.

Today, as usual, Joshua went straight for the alphabet puzzle. He tipped out the letters and quickly sequenced *a* through *g*. He reached for the *m*, the *s*, the *q*. None of them fit.

Along with deficits in language and memory, Joshua had not yet learned to formulate strategies that could help him in moments of need. I had been trying to teach him such a strategy. "When you get stuck," I reminded him, "you put your finger on the last letter and ask a question. The question is: What comes after *g*? What's the question?" Joshua repeated the question, mouthed several letters leading up to *g*, selected *h*, and moved on. The next time Joshua began grasping at random letters, I reminded him simply, "What's the question?" He asked the question aloud and located the next letter. When Joshua was unsure of what came next, I supplied the name of the letter. After completing the puzzle three times, Joshua put it back on the shelf.

We moved on to picture cards. These had become a mainstay of our language-building work. In addition to increasing the number of words in Joshua's vocabulary, I was hoping that the regularity of the format and of the work itself would help create and strengthen the memory for words that Joshua lacked.

I had found two intersecting pieces of cardboard, which we stood up and glued onto a flat base to form four rooms. These became a kitchen, a bathroom, a bedroom, and a living room. Joshua designated the living room by name; I had to elicit or supply the names of the other three rooms. The words on our picture cards had been coming from the furniture and other items that we made and added to Joshua's house. This provided a lively break from using picture dictionaries as a source of new words.

Joshua took his cards and a pencil. *Bathtub* and *sink* came to him easily. He checked them. The word *rug* did not. I offered him *r . . . ; ru . . .* He completed the word. Joshua almost remembered *blanket*, which he had cut from a scrap of fuzzy purple cloth. The word *curtains* eluded him. We opened the curtains, closed the curtains, cut out a new window and made a new pair of curtains, using the word over and over as we carried out these activities. I wanted to believe that the word was taking root, as others had.

Once we had gone over Joshua's eight or ten picture cards, we turned to the house itself. Joshua had a clear idea of what was needed, even when he could not name the item. He wanted a "thing you light" in the bedroom. We ad-libbed a lamp, glued it on top of the dresser, and made a picture card. Joshua drew a socket. We taped a string to the lamp, poked a hole in the outlet, and tied the string around a paper fastener. "Plug it in" became a new phrase for Joshua. It joined other words on that day's picture cards.

Douglas

Douglas had made significant gains in language and reading in two-and-one-half years. He was beginning to add word attack skills to his impressive stock of sight vocabulary. Douglas had begun using his newly acquired phonics knowledge to write short, predictable words from dictation. My hope was that these first steps in writing would bring him to the point of being able and willing to write his own personal stories. Several major obstacles stood in the way of this goal.

The first was handwriting. At age eight, Douglas' fine motor coordination was poorly developed, making the act of writing a chore for him. For two months, we had devoted part of every session to forming letters in a systematic and legible fashion.

The second obstacle to writing freely was Douglas' resistance to using inventive spelling. No stranger to failure, Douglas could not tolerate approximations that he knew to be wrong, even though he was unable to correct them. Deliberate misspelling also offended Douglas' strong sense of order, which had begun to serve him well in other learning situations.

Third, Douglas was just beginning to develop the phonics concepts that would eventually increase his confidence as a writer.

Even though his handwriting and phonics skills were at a very basic level, I decided to ease Douglas into meaningful writing. My hope was that engaging in writing that mattered to him would elevate our work in phonics to a real, perhaps even an urgent, need. This intuition prompted me to hang up lengths of paper on the wall for a new kind of group log. Apparently, the moment was a good one for all the children. After a labored start, their stories and mine became a daily attraction, and an inspiration for the next round of writing.

Douglas was been more or less compliant about struggling through his daily two or three sentences. His intense concentration while forming letters engendered more interest and satisfaction than the content itself. On this day, the beginning of the fifth week of the log, Douglas had come into the resource room with a copy of *The Berenstain Bears and the Stranger* (Berenstain 1985). He wanted to write about "strangers" for the log. This was the first time that the impetus for writing had come from him. I suspected he wanted to read the book with me and write about it. But I was mistaken.

Douglas picked up his pencil. I asked him to tell me his sentence before he began to write. This gave me the chance to offer help where needed, and prevent the frustration that had been a major element in Douglas' life. "One day . . . no, I mean, you know, at night, it's a little dark?" he asked. "You mean 'evening'?" Douglas nodded. I asked him if he knew how to start the word. He shook his head "no." I had a piece of scrap paper ready. At this stage, I preferred to give Douglas a word he needed, rather than burdening him with a task he found particularly difficult and exasperating. This freed Douglas enough that he was sometimes willing to risk an attempt or two on scrap paper. This time, I wrote the word.

Having heard Douglas' sentence, I knew he planned to write that one evening, Timmy and Kim's mother called them to bed. I decided not to help Douglas improve upon the sentence itself. As he wrote, I ignored his omission of "'s." The /s/ was a sound he hardly heard, and we had not yet discussed this use of apostrophes. But as Douglas was about to finish the word "call," I interrupted and asked whether this story was happening right then, or whether it had happened before, in the past. Douglas thought about it and answered "in the past." I told him he needed /ed/ at the end because that's how we know it's past. He wanted to know why and I told him "just because." He accepted it and was about to go on.

A thought struck me. Reading every other sentence had been so effective in increasing children's ease and ability as readers. I wondered whether writing alternate sentences might not lessen the burden for Douglas and enable him to express himself more fully. Sylvia Ashton-Warner (1963) described her distress at seeing pages of unrelated sentences in children's writing. She decried these "first lessons in disintegration" (p. 206). Ashton-Warner went on to say that writing "must be cohesive. An integrated, developing idea. Every word presented must be part of a grand design." I wondered whether sharing the chore of spelling and letter formation with Douglas might help him move toward a new level of writing.

"My turn," I volunteered. "You tell me the next sentence and I'll write it." An odd little smile came to Douglas' face. The offer was clearly accepted.

Douglas' chronicle of a kidnapping poured out of him. I asked him whether his story was fiction or nonfiction. He pondered the question, then told me it was both. I told him that many stories are both.

Douglas reached the end of the page. A whole page of writing was a first for him, and he was exhilarated. He had carefully monitored his handwriting throughout, cheerfully erasing now and then when a letter had not met his standards. He let me know that he intended to go on from there the next morning, and that he was writing a book.

Douglas stood up, pushed in his chair, and followed me toward the door. "Wait a minute, Ms. Stelling!" he exclaimed. He ran back, took out his writing, and at the top of the page proudly printed: "Chapter 1."

chapter 1
One evening Timmy and Kim' mother called them to bed. Their Mom said, I will bring you chocolate chip cookies and milk. At midnight the strangers came He broke the window He sneak into the house.

Chapter 2
The strangers hid in the closets. The mother turned off the lights and went to sleep. The boys went to sleep. The strangers came to the boys' room. They cover there mouth. They picked them

up, and sneaked
out the door. They
put them in the
back of the van

They drove
off When the
boys woke up, the
screamed for help
At 8:00 the mother
screamed her
boys were kid-
napped! The

neighor came over
Why are you
screaming? she
asked. The mother
went back inside
and called 911. The
police he say he
was on his way.
When he saw the
kidnappers' van,
the five other
police got in from

of the van, and
the van stopped
They got boys
When they got
the boys home,
their mother was
happy to see them
The kidnappers
went to jail!
the end

INTEGRATED LEARNING

One way of achieving a comfortable pace along with rich and varied content is to relate seemingly disparate areas to a single overall activity. Reading together has been one such opportunity. Children who are absorbed in a book are not aware that they are moving back and forth from reading to auditory training, from speechreading to writing, from vocabulary to language concepts. Children do not perceive these detours as interruptions, because they grow out of and lead back to the story.

In the same way, language skills are endowed with meaning when they enhance children's ability to express themselves in pieces of writing that matter to them. History, science, or language arts projects, discussions around a theme—any of these can serve as a living core that gives meaning and purpose to the work of developing basic skills.

FLEXIBILITY

The integrated approach has an additional benefit. Some activities can be structured so as to be flexible with regard to time. Art and poetry boxes, timelines, and information notebooks need not be addressed on a daily basis. They can be set aside and turned to as time allows. Other activities, such as book charts and literature "clubs," take only a few moments, while forming visible and cumulative records that become more informative as time goes on. All such activities provide a framework for ongoing language development, while allowing the teacher to remain available for the day-to-day demands of the classroom.

Integrated learning is a key concept of whole language. Incorporated into the resource room setting, it replaces fragmentation with coherence. A natural choice for meaning-oriented learning, it also has the effect of seeming to slow down the pace, because we are not jumping from one subject to another. Instead we are weaving a whole cloth, pulling in now one thread, now another around a central topic.

AN IDEAL WORKSPACE

Calkins (1983) reflects on the role of a simple, consistent learning environment:

> It is significant to realize that the most creative environments in our society are not the ever-changing ones. The artist's studio, the researcher's laboratory, and the scholar's library are each deliberately kept simple so as to support the complexities of the work-in-progress. They are deliberately kept predictable, so the unpredictable can happen (p. 32).

In the resource room, this has meant:

- storing material in an orderly and systematic way;
- keeping material in current use easily accessible;
- rearranging books, supplies, material, and furniture periodically to reflect children's changing needs;
- passing along or discarding material that is no longer useful; and
- keeping the resource room as uncluttered and visually pleasing as possible.

The physical environment influences, to a degree, the nature and structure of the resource room day. When Curtis and I set out to read *The Chalkbox Kid*, the resource room was housed in a bright and spacious room. Baskets of books lined the walls and occupied a free-standing shelving unit. Books were sorted into categories: dictionaries, picture books, folk and fairy tales, mysteries, novels, science, history, biographies, anthologies, poetry, and books of general information. Among the works of fiction were sets of books by particular authors. Stories with cassettes filled a box on an unused desk across from a bin of art books. Baskets were labeled. There was ample space for children to approach each area freely and to browse comfortably.

A wall-length bulletin board as well as a wall-length blackboard provided space for works in progress. These included reading and writing logs and phonics envelopes; Authors Club, Illustrators Club, and Theme Club forms; vocabulary hundred-squares, a world map, and more.

The size of the room allowed for two work spaces: a large table and chairs for the older children, and a small table and chairs for the younger ones. This helped make the resource room period comfortable for all.

A CHANGE OF LOCATION

At some point, it became necessary to give up our resource room "home" to a colleague whose need for space was greater than ours. Our new location was a long, narrow paper closet in active use. At the far end, the closet broadened out enough to accommodate a low table and several small chairs. By rearranging some of the paper and supplies, I was able to clear away a number of shelves for our own use. All of the book baskets fit neatly onto the shelves on one side of the table. As before, they looked cheerfully inviting.

To my disappointment, the children took little notice of our resource room library in its new surroundings. The same books that had been perused, signed out, read at home and in school, and exchanged for new selections were now little more than ornamental. I mulled over the children's ages, their levels, their self-motivation, and my own role in inspiring them to read. The answer turned out to be far simpler: there was not enough space for children to fit comfortably between the table and the shelves. No wonder they did not gravitate toward the book baskets.

A time factor also entered into the picture. In our former room, children had socialized with one another and pored over books while I checked the FM units in the morning and collected them at the end of the day. Because our closet had no outlet, the FM units had to be kept in an area that did not belong to us. Circumstances required that the children keep their talking to a minimum in this shared space. The beginning and end of the day lost their social and literary value. We were left with a wealth of books so close as to be beyond reach.

In place of generous expanses of blackboards and bulletin boards, our new room had only a short stretch of wall uninterrupted by shelving. On that wall we taped up vocabulary hundred-squares, our weekly group log consisting of a strip for each child and one for myself, and the children's audiograms. These were clustered around a mock audiometer, whose dial children could turn to correspond to their own hearing levels at low, medium, and high frequencies. No further space was available for work or display purposes.

BEYOND SURROUNDINGS

A closet has obvious disadvantages, both practical and aesthetic, in comparison with an airy and spacious room. The volume of reading that had taken place once children broke the reading barrier was largely a product of their daily access to an abundance of books. This situation did not prevail in the closet. Yet Joshua's modest but significant gains in language and memory took place in these cramped quarters. The seeds of focusing and concentration, which had begun with handwriting and branched out to reading, writing, and discussion, were sown for Robert as we sat in too-small chairs at a too-low table. Cathy's metamorphosis into a reader and Douglas' into a writer came about in this space, so lacking in visual appeal.

As a teacher, I have experienced discouragement and frustration, satisfaction and exhilarating discoveries in both settings. I am keenly aware of the social and educational implications of a spacious and well-lighted room. I would be reluctant to part with such a space. Yet the space itself has proven to be less crucial than the quality of teaching and learning that takes place within its walls. Ultimately, it is the partnership between teacher and child, and the absorption of both in the learning at hand, that endow the resource room setting with life and meaning.

Chapter 22

Examining "Inclusion"

This chapter addresses resource room programming for children who are deaf and hard of hearing. The chapter takes a stand in favor of retaining pull-out programs (see p. 6) as one option in the continuum of services available to children with hearing impairments. The validity of resource room placement for some children becomes particularly pointed at a time when "push-in" programs are gaining widespread acceptance.

THE IDEA

The Individuals with Disabilities Education Act or IDEA (Code of Federal Regulations 1993) came into being in 1975 to protect the civil rights of children with handicapping conditions. At this time, only about 50% of children with special needs were receiving appropriate educational services.

The IDEA mandates that every child be provided with a "free appropriate public education." The most appropriate placement is understood to be the "least restrictive environment" in which a child can grow socially, emotionally, and academically. The least restrictive environment most closely approximates the school and class the child would be attending if he or she had no disability.

The IDEA gives children with disabilities the right to be educated with children who are nondisabled to the maximum extent appropriate. Special classes and separate schools are provided for children whose disabilities are so severe that they are unable to benefit from regular class placement even with support services.

ISSUES SPECIFIC TO DEAF AND HARD-OF-HEARING CHILDREN

Ross et al. (1991) emphasize that "hearing-impaired children should be educated in those places that offer them the greatest opportunities—psychosocial, academic, and communicative—and cause the least disruption to the integrity of the family unit" (p. 1). For some children, the so-called least restrictive environment is not necessarily the most appropriate school placement. For others, general education with support services provides both the least restrictive and the most appropriate educational setting.

Advocates of mainstreaming for children who are deaf and hard of hearing, like advocates for inclusion in general, believe that children gain from a setting that reflects the diversity of regular school and community life. They believe that children benefit from the relatively higher expectations of the mainstream curriculum, in contrast to the typically more modest expectations of separate settings. Advocates of mainstreaming believe that learning to socialize and to manage their disabilities in the school setting prepares children for participation in everyday life outside of school as well.

Those who favor separate schools and settings, on the other hand, point to deafness as a unique human experience. They believe strongly that schools and classes designed for deaf children maximize social interaction and promote the language and traditions of Deaf culture.

For hearing-impaired children, as for all children with disabilities, regular class placement with some form of supplementary support constitutes a choice in the federally mandated range of options. In summarizing a series of interviews with deaf adults educated in a variety of settings, Foster (1989) notes advantages and disadvantages inherent in each setting. Whatever their conviction, parents and educators support the primacy of choice for individual families.

THE NEED FOR FLEXIBILITY

Because children have different needs at different times, the flexibility that allows children to move from one option to another is more important than the advantages of any one program. A child such as Cathy (see Chapters 18 and 21) exemplifies the need for reconsidering children's placement based upon reassessment of their needs and abilities.

Cathy entered kindergarten in her neighborhood school. When her hearing loss was identified at age seven, she began to receive support services from an itinerant teacher who worked with her several times a week. By third grade, it was becoming clear that Cathy needed more intensive remediation than this situation could offer. She was reevaluated and placed in the resource room program, where she repeated third grade.

During that year, Cathy's language developed somewhat, and she began to acquire a foundation in reading. However, her difficulty with the pace, volume of work, and teaching style of the regular class made it clear that she needed a more controlled learning environment. Cathy was evaluated again and placed in a self-contained class for children with learning disorders, along with continued resource room support.

Cathy responded well to this combination. At the end of sixth grade, she came close to achieving a grade-level reading score. At that point, she was evaluated once more and decertified from special education. Cathy entered a junior high school "inclusion class," team-taught by one regular and one special education teacher. An itinerant teacher met with Cathy several times a week to continue work on language development, and to help Cathy keep up with class assignments.

INTEGRATION AND MAINSTREAMING:
TWO POSSIBILITIES

The integrated classroom allows children with disabilities to learn at their own pace and level along with their nondisabled peers. In one such model, classroom teachers are regarded as "preexisting natural supports" (York and Vandercook 1989) while the special education teacher is to be "faded" whenever appropriate, so that the child's classmates and classroom teacher can acquire the skills they need to foster interaction and independence.

The authors describe a second-grade girl whose Individualized Educational Plan (IEP) included such goals as maintaining a supported sitting position, using picture cues to select an audiotape, and turning the pages of a book as a peer reads aloud. Reading time provided the opportunity for her to practice depressing a switch to turn on a tape recorder. Working with class-mates to develop an essential motor skill in an age-appropriate, regular education setting was a constructive use of the reading pe-riod for this little girl with multiple handicaps, and could not have been accomplished more effectively in any other setting.

With understanding adults as role models, children prove themselves capable of accepting and encouraging a severely disabled classmate's steps toward socialization. They can be helped to understand "that Todd talks with his eyes and that Shawn communicates with his smiles and tears" (Casanave 1991, 40).

Unlike the children described above, children who are mainstreamed are capable of achieving at or near the level of their peers in general education classrooms. To meet this goal, instruction may need to be modified or adapted. The children depicted throughout *The Words They Need* are mainstreamed in regular education classes with resource room support.

A RANGE OF OPTIONS

Diverse approaches have been developed to meet the needs of children with disabilities in general education settings.

- *Team Teaching:* Regular and special educators collaborate in planning and implementing instruction for the benefit of all children. In some settings, children are not pulled out, nor is remedial instruction provided in the class-room.
- *Consulting Teachers:* Outside consultants guide classroom teachers in meeting the needs of children with handicap-ping conditions. They may prepare instructional material, select and train peer tutors (Jenkins and Jenkins 1981), and group students so as to ensure positive interaction in a cooperative learning situation (Johnson et al. 1984).
- *Paraprofessionals and Volunteers:* The services of these teaching assistants enable some children to succeed in a regular education environment.
- *Pull-Out Programs:* Students receive supplementary in-struction from a remedial teacher in a separate location. Teachers may work toward meeting classroom goals, or they may establish individual goals based on diagnostic evaluations of children's needs.

- *Push-In Programs:* Supplementary instruction takes place in the regular classroom. Special educators may be involved in a team-teaching approach designed to meet the needs of all the children in the class; or they may work with small groups that include the children with disabilities (Meyers et al. 1991).

The above options differ with regard to the nature and extent of remedial instruction offered to children with disabilities in regular classrooms. Because of the impact of hearing loss on language development, programs that minimize or eliminate direct remediation are not likely to meet the needs of mainstreamed hearing-impaired children.

THE MAINSTREAMED HEARING-IMPAIRED CHILD

The language and learning needs of deaf and hard-of-hearing children challenge even experienced, specially trained teachers. Meeting these needs is not a quick or easy process. The classroom teacher contributes to the language development of the mainstreamed hearing-impaired child; however, the diagnostic and prescriptive instruction essential to remediating severe language deficits cannot be provided by the classroom teacher. Neither can it be provided by peer tutors, even those who have been trained to place learners in an instructional sequence, deliver direct instruction, confirm correct responses, provide appropriate reinforcement, collect daily performance data, and chart and measure children's progress (Jenkins and Jenkins 1981).

A child who is deaf or hard of hearing derives the same satisfaction as his or her classmates from collaborating with an older or younger "buddy" in writing and illustrating a story based on a shared experience. The same child may solidify a phonics or computation skill with the help of a classmate who is comfortably familiar with the material. Yet neither of these situations provides the one-to-one instruction that Bloom (1984) deems the most powerful intervention for improving academic performance. Such intervention cannot be reduced to rote training, but demands a high degree of skill, knowledge, and sensitivity.

RESOURCE ROOM: ONE POSSIBILITY

Present advances in cochlear implants and other technology, coupled with early identification and intervention, make it possible for some children with hearing impairments to enter mainstream settings with age-appropriate academic and social skills.

Even when deaf and hard-of-hearing children are well prepared for participation in general education classes, some form of support is likely to be a key factor in their continued academic and social well-being. Huefner (1988) observes that consulting services "often will not substitute for more intensive intervention [and] should not replace the resource room as a primary service delivery system. . . . The resource room may well be the option of choice for genuinely handicapped students" (p. 407). For children with language needs affecting every area of learning, the resource room can provide the language remediation and development that make mainstreaming feasible.

Listening—literally and figuratively—for what each child needs requires an environment as free as possible from competing demands. Under optimal conditions, the resource room setting is relatively free from auditory and visual distractions. This affords teacher and child the time and space they need to find common ground and engage in the kinds of dialogue from which language and learning grow. The resource room teacher links current learning to previous knowledge with full cognizance of the child's language level, cognitive abilities, and emotional needs.

As communication skills grow, children may continue to experience gaps in understanding classroom presentations and discussion. Ongoing classroom observation, as well as communication with classroom teachers, alert the resource room teacher to learning needs related to language and curriculum. Problems specific to the hearing-impaired child can then be addressed in the resource room. "Preteaching," a strategy for increasing children's ability to comprehend and participate in classroom lessons, is described in Chapter 2.

The children in my own experience typically enter the resource room having achieved few of the commonly acknowledged prerequisites for successful mainstreaming. (See Chapter 2 for mainstreaming criteria.) Significant deficits coupled with intense remediation have resulted in atypical learning profiles: a child may make progress in areas directly addressed in the resource room, while lagging behind in other areas. At the same time, developing any ability often serves to strengthen others. The achievements of many children by the end of elementary school attest to their growth in the mainstream program. Some go on to approach or achieve grade level in junior high, others in high school. In retrospect, their accomplishments justify considering regular class placement for some children who do not meet commonly held criteria for successful mainstreaming.

PULL-OUT OR PUSH-IN?

The question arises as to whether a special education service such as resource room support ought to be confined to the resource room or brought into the classroom setting in the interest of maximum integration.

Pull-out programs have been criticized for:

- minimizing classroom teachers' responsibility for instruction;
- not having adequate collaboration between classroom and resource room teachers;
- segregating children unnecessarily;
- fragmenting the curriculum;
- reducing time on task; and
- causing the stigma associated with receiving resource room services (Meyers et al. 1991).

Push-in programs have corresponding disadvantages.

- Typical school schedules allow classroom and support teachers little joint planning time to create small-group activities designed to take place at the same time as whole-class instruction and work toward meeting the same goals.
- Lack of space in overcrowded classrooms may make it difficult for the resource room teacher to work with a small group that includes the child with a hearing impairment.
- Small-group activities conducted against a background of whole-class or other small-group lessons can be distracting not only to the children involved, but to other children in the class who have difficulty focusing under those circumstances.

Both pull-out and push-in programs contain advantages and disadvantages. Stigma and social constraints may be issues for some children in either setting. Planning and scheduling difficulties are inherent in both programs. My experience with children who manifest significant language deficits at a fundamental level has led to an appreciation of what can be accomplished in the resource room setting. My own conviction is that the learning potential of hearing-impaired children such as these is best achieved with the help of a consistent and intensive course of remediation in the resource room itself.

Children whose remedial teacher comes into the classroom remain present for the full flow of social and instructional activities. For children whose class participation is still limited by language deficits, however, remedial work will necessarily differ in pace and content from the work of the class. This apparent fragmentation is unavoidable in the early stages of language development. Though missing class time while in the resource room, children are building skills that will eventually make time spent on classroom tasks profitable and worthwhile.

Meyers et al. (1991) view push-in programs as "reducing the distinctiveness of classroom and specialist teacher's roles" (p. 8). For deaf and hard-of-hearing children with language delays, it is the distinctive roles of the resource room and resource room teacher that help make classroom learning possible.

NO TIME TO LOSE

Macdonald and York (1989) note that nonsubject areas may actually be the most important for integrated students with disabilities. Casanave (1991) describes the interactions between Andrew and his friends as they eat lunch, play together on the playground, and sit next to each other at story time. Shared activities such as these represent fulfilling life experiences for this eight-year-old boy with mental retardation and his third-grade classmates.

Deaf and hard-of-hearing resource room children are already mainstreamed. For them, achieving a satisfying life to the fullest extent possible has a major academic component. Grade-level achievement becomes a realistic goal as language is systematically developed. Deaf and hard-of-hearing doctors and lawyers, educators and scientists, actors and actresses, authors, social workers, dancers, and others attest to the potential of this group of children.

It is imperative that children who are deaf and hard of hearing be helped to make up for lost time as quickly as possible. Only by providing unique conditions for meeting their needs can the resource room justify the inconvenience posed by the pull-out aspects of the program.

- The resource room setting enables the teacher to diagnose and meet hearing- and language-related needs with maximum efficiency.
- Teacher and child can work in a structured and highly focused way on a purposeful sequence of interrelated activities that further underlying goals.
- The teacher is free to link learning with class activities or not, according to children's needs.

For children who have missed so much, the resource room is a haven. Learning is made accessible, enabling children to use their minds and discover their own intelligence, often for the first time.

THE LANGUAGE OF POSSIBILITY

As children approach the point of full class participation, working in the classroom allows the remedial teacher to help them apply their knowledge and skills to the work of the class. This may involve organization, following directions, and developing strategies for class participation.

Reaching this point presupposes a thorough grounding in basic language and academic skills. Developing these skills is the responsibility and obligation of the resource room teacher. In so doing, he or she prepares children to take their place in the mainstream and benefit from all that regular education has to offer.

Capper (1989) speaks of leaders in education who can "articulate the language of possibility" for even the most severely disabled students (p. 2). The resource room setting helps make the language of possibility a reality for mainstreamed deaf and hard-of-hearing children.

Chapter 23

Educational Research

Along with teaching, there is another discipline dedicated to gaining insight into how children learn. This is educational research. Becoming familiar with the work of researchers is valuable to teachers in two ways.

- It corroborates and affirms and/or challenges our own observations and experience.
- It offers fresh ways of looking at the teaching-learning process.

The following researchers have examined the development of language and reading. Some have focused on students learning English as a second language, others on children in general. The issues they address are germane to the education of children who are deaf and hard of hearing.

LANGUAGE AND COMMUNICATION

Jerome Bruner (1978) emphasizes the social nature of language acquisition. He contends that language lacks vitality when taught as a separate subject. Language takes on life as a means of communication about content of interest.

Bruner believes that linguistic development is impeded when written activities predominate and the teacher does most of the talking. He has found that environments that are low in anxiety and high in interest are more conducive to language development.

Bruner regards the study of correct language as useful, as long as it serves the language acquisition process and does not become an end in itself.

Merrill Swain (1985), like Bruner, emphasizes that using language interactively is essential to the language acquisition process. Swain's point of view is that confirmation checks and other feedback from a competent speaker provide children with the impetus and guidance they need to get their meaning across more clearly. Without feedback, children have no way of progressing beyond their own limited strategies for making themselves understood.

LANGUAGE AND MEANING

Margaret Donaldson (1978) notes that young children's language develops within a clear and predictable contextual framework. Language used by young children, and by adults speaking to young children, is almost secondary to the obvious clues inherent in the situation. Donaldson refers to this as "embedded" thought and language, in that both are embedded in the immediate context.

Donaldson cautions that children's facility in producing language tied to the situation at hand may be misleading. It is not necessarily indicative of language skills in a broader sense. When children use language, they are in control. They choose what they want to talk about, and are free to interpret the situation in their own way.

As thinking and language move beyond meaningful interpersonal contexts, new demands are created. The child now needs to focus on "disembedded" linguistic forms, rather than on situational cues. This happens when the child becomes the listener, and occurs in kindergarten, if not before.

According to Donaldson, children manifest much higher levels of cognitive ability when tasks are presented in an embedded context, or one that is related to children's own experiences. She argues that disembedding early instruction in reading and other areas from children's out-of-school experiences contributes significantly to children's educational difficulties.

SOME ROLES OF INSTRUCTION IN LANGUAGE DEVELOPMENT

Piaget's "readiness" theory formulates that maturation precedes learning. Concepts develop spontaneously as children mature. Teacher input must be kept comfortably within the child's level.

Lev Vygotsky (1962), in contrast, speaks of two distinct levels of development:

- the "actual developmental level" as determined by the child's ability to solve problems independently; and
- the "potential developmental level" as determined by the child's problem-solving ability with guidance.

Vygotsky proposes that instruction is a powerful source of concepts. Through instruction, the child's potential developmental level can become his or her next actual developmental level. Vygotsky names the distance between what has been achieved and what can be attained with guidance the "Zone of Proximal Development." The bridge is crossed when "the teacher, in dialogue with the student, focuses on emerging skills and abilities" (p. 33).

According to Vygotsky, teaching within the child's actual developmental level limits learning to what the child can already do. The only worthwhile instruction "marches ahead of development and leads it" (p. 188).

Understanding Vygotsky's point of view helps us to delineate the child's immediate learning needs and to work dynamically on those areas that are in the course of maturing.

Rod Ellis (1985) also views the teacher as guide. Teachers help students make their way in a language that still poses many obstacles. Ellis asserts that language learners need many opportunities to understand and make themselves understood in a variety of situations. He concludes that language develops best through natural and informal discourse with a partner who has more linguistic resources than the learner.

Ellis acknowledges motivation and personality as factors in language acquisition.

Michael Breene and **Christopher Candlin** (1980) join with Vygotsky and Ellis in emphasizing the interactional nature of learning. In their eyes, the shape and flow of learning grow out of the interaction between learners, teachers, texts, and activities.

It is by keeping curriculum and content flexible that teachers preserve the freedom to exploit children's learning and give shape to it in ways that make language acquisition most likely.

Breene and Candlin emphasize that, as curriculum designers, we cannot predict with certainty the level of learning that will evolve in a learning situation. All we can do is "anticipate a range of content which will richly activate learning competencies so that the ultimate target repertoire becomes accessible and its specific demands recognized by the learner" (p. 103).

Toward this end, teachers need to ensure that content is significant to students in both the cognitive and the affective domains. The state of the learner will then suggest the learning sequence. Throughout this process, it is the teacher who:

- facilitates communication between children;
- facilitates communication between children and activities;
- acts as an interdependent participant within the teaching-learning group;
- organizes resources;
- is herself or himself a resource; and
- acts as a guide in the sense of offering and seeking feedback at appropriate moments.

LANGUAGE AND CLARITY

Stephen Krashen (1982) notes the difficulties that second-language learners face when assaulted by a barrage of incomprehensible language. Teachers can make language comprehensible by keeping in mind ways in which the primary language was learned at an earlier age. Krashen advises teachers to employ:

- short, simple sentences;
- high-frequency vocabulary;
- "here and now" items related to the immediate situation;
- frequent gesture;
- indirect correction;
- lack of overt attention to form; and
- comprehension checks.

Krashen maintains that students acquire language when messages of real interest and relevance are transmitted and understood. He suggests working on communication at a point a bit beyond the student's own level. Teacher-input needs to contain structures that the learner has not yet acquired, but is "ready" for.

LANGUAGE AND READING

Frank Smith (1985) believes that the key to reading with comprehension resides not in the text, but in the linguistic and experiential background of the reader. In order to read, children must be equipped with:

- an understanding of relevant language;
- familiarity with the subject matter; and
- some general reading ability.

Smith distinguishes between visual information and general information. Printed letters and words constitute visual information. General information consists of language and background knowledge. Smith believes the sounding out of words to be of secondary importance. Reading with comprehension requires the language and background information that take place "behind the eyes." Smith advocates teaching reading through whole words and context clues, with phonics playing a minor, supporting role.

Smith addresses the needs of remedial students. He maintains that the most effective means of helping children in difficulty is to show them that reading is not a painful or a pointless academic exercise, and that learning to read is well within their grasp. The first step is to select interesting reading material, and to help children become familiar with the language of books. Collaborative reading is a means toward this end, and a path toward independent reading. It provides the reassurance that, in Smith's eyes, is a basis of remedial instruction.

John Oller (1983) is concerned with the kind of reading material that best promotes language acquisition.

According to Oller, we take note of our experience and remember it in what he calls "episodic form." The two ingredients of episodic form are logic and conflict.

- A sequence of events feels logical if one action leads to another in a way that is consistent with our own everyday experience. We understand and are likely to remember a logical sequence because it makes sense.
- Conflict or tension gives shape to events and speaks to our emotions.

Reading material that contains logic and conflict is true to life and appeals to both our intellects and our emotions. Oller believes that grammar books can be useful if supplemental in nature, but that texts consisting of unrelated sentences have no intrinsic meaning or appeal.

The following examples, first of unrelated sentences and then of related ones, are taken from Richard-Amato (1996, 285–86).

Example 1:

1. We're having a grammar test today.
2. Bob is having a party tomorrow.
3. The Smith's are having a good time in Paris.

Questions related to this exercise are impossible to answer without referring back to the text because:

- the people are not important to us and do not connect to each other in any meaningful way;
- they are not part of any conflict and thus remain unmotivated (have no reason for their actions); and
- they make little impression and are not easily remembered.

Example 2:

Darlene: I think I'll call Bettina's mother. It's almost five and Chrissy isn't home yet.

Meg: I thought Bettina had the chicken pox.

Darlene: Oh, that's right. I forgot. Chrissy didn't go to Bettina's today. Where is she?

We are more likely to remember details from this passage. Its structure is consistent with our own experience. The dialogue is motivated and logical. We become concerned with the little girl's disappearance just as the people in the story are concerned. We become involved at both conscious and subconscious levels.

Oller lists some implications of his "Episodic Hypothesis" for classroom teaching.

- Unmotivated texts should be avoided.
- The story line should be carried primarily by stageable action (it should be possible to dramatize the story.)
- Basic facts must be understood before the student can be expected to understand the subtleties.
- The story can be broken down into manageable "chunks" for a better grasp of the facts.
- Each episode can be worked through in multiple cycles, from simple to complex.
- Children progress from basic facts to more in-depth understanding.

Stories that engage our intellect and our emotions are, almost by definition, of literary merit. This is the reading Oller proposes if we are to inspire children to acquire language through reading.

SUMMARY

Children who are deaf and hard of hearing share the needs of all children with regard to conditions that promote language learning. Miller and Luckner (1992) cite surveys which estimate that teachers account for 75% of classroom communication. This statistic holds true for teachers of the deaf as well. The authors, themselves teachers of the deaf, remind us that children learn language by engaging in conversation in a multitude of settings for a variety of purposes. They urge educators to shift their emphasis from teaching language to facilitating language. This happens when we collaborate with students in helping them to communicate their messages more effectively.

Like Miller and Luckner, the researchers summarized in this chapter emphasize the interactive nature of communication. They stress the need for language learning to be structured around content of compelling personal interest. Teachers of children who are deaf and hard of hearing need, in addition, to build a foundation of experience and background knowledge as prerequisites for further learning.

This is what all children need if they are to capitalize on their ability to acquire language. This is what deaf and hard-of-hearing children need as they reach past vocabulary and syntax to language mastery.

Chapter 24

In Search of "Relevance"

Over and over, researchers and educators alike stress the importance of making language activities meaningful to the learner. My experience has been that attempts to create relevance by such means as reducing learning tasks to comic book format imply a superficial understanding of the concept of relevance. True relevance entails helping children stretch their skills and intellects to meet new challenges.

ASPECTS OF RELEVANCE

What constitutes "relevance," and how can we bring learning into the realm of significance for children?

Oller (1983) specifies three conditions needed if "input" is to become "intake":

- adequate language development;
- sufficient knowledge; and
- maturation of the child's ability to make sense of the experience (p. 6).

To meet these conditions, we lay the language and informational groundwork basic to each new learning task, then aim a bit beyond in order to bring the child forward in each of these areas. We make sure that what we are asking of the child is within the range of his or her language, knowledge, and maturity levels.

At this critical juncture, how can we increase the likelihood that children will take what is being offered and make it their own? Oller finds the answer in establishing a link between language and experience. This is fundamental resource room practice.

- A simple identification can provide the steppingstone to broader learning. Recognizing George Washington on a dollar bill and taping it to the timeline under Colonial Times was all that was needed to ease John into a picture biography of the first president (see p. 162). The book, at first foreign and overwhelming, became a cheerful continuation of something comfortably familiar.
- The linking may be more complex. Cathy expressed a wish to make some gilded dried flowers like those she had bought as a gift. Weeks later, the classroom teacher assigned a report on the stock market. Planning the production of the flowers, and discussing how to fund materials and an assistant, paved the way to understanding basic concepts related to the stock market.

Learning acquires significance when not-yet familiar information evolves out of prior knowledge. The new knowledge, in turn, becomes part of the child's ever-widening knowledge base. Kagan (1968) views prior learning as a prerequisite to sustained involvement. Engagement with learning is an outward sign that children are finding answers to their own intellectual needs. This meeting between mind and learning task is relevance made visible.

Self-Esteem: A Detour

Educator Lilian Katz (1993) proposes that children gain in self-respect when provided with "challenging opportunities to build self-confidence through effort, persistence, and the gradual accrual of skills, knowledge, and appropriate behavior" (p. 21).

Katz discredits exercises such as "I am special because. . . ." In her opinion, activities designed to help children feel good about themselves cross the line from self-respect to self-preoccupation. Like stars, stickers, and empty praise, they express a limited understanding of self-esteem.

In their place, Katz values an appreciation of children's interests and efforts in the learning sphere. By deepening interest in learning itself, teachers provide positive feedback "without deflecting children from the content" (pp. 22–23).

Lerner (1996) distinguishes between "feel-good-now" self-esteem and "earned" self-esteem. I have seen children slowly acquire skills and abilities that have led to pride and pleasure in their accomplishments. My part has been to structure individual activities and the overall progression of learning in such a way that learning tasks, while challenging, do not become frustratingly difficult. The knowledge that they can depend on this support and guidance has enabled some children to persist in their efforts.

Earned self-esteem is hard won. Children's motivation and satisfaction grow out of their immersion in learning. The children with whom I have worked have not had the preparation required to participate fully in mainstream classes early in their school lives. Perhaps for this reason, I have sometimes detected signs of growing competence long before the children themselves have begun to perceive themselves as capable learners. When that moment comes, competence and confidence combine, and learning moves forward with new vigor.

Relevance and Self-Esteem: Unexpected Partners

Kagan (1968) reminds us that we need to prepare children to wonder (p. 87). Otherwise, the most enticing object or situation will capture their interest only momentarily. Kagan ascribes disinterest and lack of curiosity to a lack of preparation for the experience at hand. Bringing to light a connection between unfamiliar material and something within children's experience is an important kind of preparation. Children feel empowered as they become aware of their own knowledge. This feeling of mastery engenders the confidence that sparks further interest.

Relevance and self-esteem combine when new learning grows out of previous experience. Tasks that may have felt abstract and overwhelming become a logical and inviting extension of what the child already knows. It is this kind of meaning that makes real learning possible, and it is learning that engenders genuine and lasting self-esteem.

Chapter 25

Teaching and Learning: A Complex Dynamic

> *In homes where role models do not stimulate the child, where conversations, questions, and reading are not encouraged, the child enters school short on basic tools. He will ask fewer questions, use shorter sentences, have a smaller vocabulary and a shorter attention span than his more advantaged classmates.*
>
> *Trelease 1985, 17*

The effectiveness of early intervention programs for young hearing-impaired children depends on the extent to which parents link language learning to the activities of daily living. Engaging children in preverbal play lays the foundation for communication. Creating a predictable environment engenders routines to which children can attach basic language. The carefully paced introduction of challenging situations stimulates the development of new knowledge and abilities. Early and consistent amplification enables children to interpret what they hear to the maximum extent possible. For an in-depth discussion of parental involvement and the early language development of hearing-impaired children, see Boothroyd (1988).

Meeting the needs of young children presents challenges to all parents. Parents of hearing-impaired infants, toddlers, and preschoolers face the task of helping their children develop language with a minimum of feedback to guide them. Speech and language programs offer guidance in taking advantage of learning opportunities in everyday life. As parents gain confidence in tailoring learning experiences to their child's existing skills and abilities, language and communication grow.

Not all families possess the time and abilities needed for systematic language stimulation. Few of the parents in *The Words They Need* have had the support of a speech and language program. Long working hours, difficult family situations, and a variety of personal circumstances have deprived these parents of the time and energy they might otherwise have brought to meeting the needs of their deaf and hard-of-hearing children.

A child whose parents take an active part in his or her language development may well reach school age able to participate in class activities with a moderate amount of resource room or other support and a minimum of adjustment on the part of the classroom teacher. In contrast, what can we expect of ourselves and of our teaching as we work with those children who are ill-prepared for the demands of regular classes, even with resource room assistance, and whose parents are less capable of playing a role in their children's education? What can we hope for children who lack exposure to language and learning, who suffer from sensory and experiential deprivation, whose hearing loss may be compounded by educational neglect?

WHAT TEACHERS CAN DO

As teachers of deaf and hard-of-hearing children at all language levels, we are challenged to find our own responses to individual needs. Just as Sylvia Ashton-Warner treasured words that gave voice to children's deepest feelings and discarded those that did not, we, too, are free to pick and choose among various possibilities in our own teaching. As we work, the experience of fellow educators can point the way to further reading, writing, and language competence.

As we teach, we offer our children the best of our knowledge, experience, judgment, and intuition.

- We give them a grounding in oral and written language, reading, and general information. We guide them in progressing in each area to the extent that time, and their own capacities and motivation, allow.
- We observe children carefully, looking for clues that will help us understand our students as children and as learners.
- "We can't give the children rich lives, but we can give them the lens to appreciate the richness that is already in their lives" (Calkins 1991, 35). As we uncover the uniqueness of each child's character and life experience, we re-

flect this back in a way that opens children's eyes to self-discovery and self-esteem.

- We engage children's participation by making learning experiences relevant and attainable so that children feel safe in attempting them.
- We offer children that "bonded relationship with a joyfully literate adult" (Calkins 1991, 239) which is the key to inspiring a love of reading and writing.
- We lift schoolwork out of the humdrum and endow learning moments with meaning.

ADDITIONAL FACTORS

Factors beyond our control have a powerful impact on children's ability to learn. Being deaf or hard of hearing does not protect children against circumstances that make learning difficult for any child. When Caldecott Medal winner Gail Haley pleaded that "children who are not spoken to by live and responsive adults will not learn to speak properly" and that "children who are not read to will have few reasons for wanting to learn to read" (p. 225), she was addressing the needs of all children. Children who are deaf and hard of hearing may not be spoken to or read to because they lack adequate language for comprehension at their age level. A persistent lack of stimulation can then exacerbate their problems in acquiring language.

Lucy Calkins (1991) reminisces about a childhood bursting with the intensity and engagement that accompanied projects such as building a dam across a creek or organizing a neighborhood pet show. To Calkins, this blurring of the line between work and play, between imagination and industriousness, has its roots in childhood and continues to characterize learning at its best. Like all children, deaf and hard-of-hearing children who go from school to after-school programs, from baby-sitters to tired working parents lose a precious part of their childhood with each missed opportunity for experiences such as these.

When asked what happened to the classics as suggested read-alouds, Jim Trelease (1985) replied that "nothing happened to the classics—but something happened to children: their imaginations went to sleep in front of the television 25 years ago" (p. 75).

In *The Plug-In Drug* (1985), Marie Winn maintains that the greater the child's verbal opportunities, the greater the likelihood that his language will grow in complexity and that his rational, verbal thinking abilities will sharpen. In contrast, as children passively absorb television words and images hour after hour, day after day with little mental effort, a pattern emphasizing nonverbal cognition becomes established. Deaf and hard-of-hearing children, along with others, have had their imaginations and language stunted by this fact of modern life.

HOW FAR CAN WE GO?

Sylvia Ashton-Warner (1963) believed that her role as a teacher was to call on the child's own resources. For this, she needed the patience and wisdom to listen, to watch, and to wait until the child's line of thought became apparent.

Resource room children require more explicit teaching. At the same time, Ashton-Warner is saying something important. As teachers, we are not the only variables in the teaching-learning equation. Along with other factors beyond our control, the child's motivation enters into it very early. An 18-month-old toddler in a speech therapy session who bangs on the table between activities as if to say "Let's go!" is demonstrating a will to learn. At any age, a child can display self-motivation or need to be carried along.

Brackett (1990) maintains that students should be held accountable for practicing and refining the specific skills that have been introduced to them. It is the students' responsibility to make themselves understood by monitoring their own communication and adapting it to the listener's level. It is up to the students to incorporate methods of language expansion into their own communication.

"All that parents and teachers can do for their child," observed Anne Sullivan, "is to surround that child with the right conditions. The child will do the rest; the things she will do for herself are the only things that really count in education" (in Calkins 1991, 291).

We teach, adjust, reflect, teach, adjust, and reflect again. One child becomes a motivated partner in the learning process; another does not. How can we give ourselves what we need to sustain this difficult and sometimes draining effort, in ways that keep us fresh for our own sake and that of our children?

Putting Ourselves First

As teachers, we enjoy and appreciate individual differences in children. We deserve to accord ourselves the same respect. We can do this by finding ways of working that feed and are fed by our own particular strengths and interests.

Lucy Calkins expressed this in a compelling way at a Writing Project conference when she exhorted educators to teach at the frontiers of their own learning. Only by responding to children's needs in ways that fascinate and excite us, can we satisfy our own needs as intelligent adults. Our aliveness to learning is the best invitation we can offer children to open their eyes to the world around and inside them.

Personalizing Our Teaching

Each of us travels a different road to this end. Because I feel more comfortable with smaller rather than larger groups, I have never achieved the lively group lessons and exchanges at which some teachers excel. I have little patience for repetitive activities such as calendar work, which in another teacher's hands may play a major role in orienting children and laying the foundation for language development. On the other hand, I feel stimulated by the challenge of identifying a word or concept that will make a child's eyes light up and become his or her own, and so I structure my teaching around that ideal. One of my interests related to working with young children has been children's literature. This has made teaching language through reading a natural inclination for me.

Smith College Teaching Award winner Margaret Cormack reflects on her own evolution as a teacher (Sheirer 1993):

> When I reached graduate school, I was able to watch my teachers very closely to see what worked for them. In fact, the teachers whom I admired the most were the ones whose style was the opposite of mine as it has developed. They were extremely organized and could give these beautiful, erudite lectures, whereas my style is to present a lot of alternatives and let the students hash them out. But I've found that you cannot adopt a style that is alien to your personality. By not trying to be somebody else, I think I get better results (p. 12).

Fellow educators have much to contribute to our understanding. Self-knowledge is crucial to making use of the experience of others. The more aware we are of our own styles and preferences as teachers, the closer we can come to recognizing in other people's work something that may work for us.

Teachers As Learners

The art of teaching, like the art of writing, demands that we step back from our work in order to reflect, ask questions, and let our insights grow.

As we examine our teaching experiences, we become conscious of what has succeeded or not succeeded, and why. This expands our capacity to diagnose children's learning needs, and to respond to them prescriptively and creatively.

In reflecting on our work, we enter the world of learners. Here we gain both expertise and humility. Working alongside children as fellow-learners is a basic tenet of the whole language philosophy. Each learning experience of our own sharpens our ability to diagnose obstacles to learning as they arise in the resource room. We empathize more easily with children's struggles to master difficult skills and concepts. We gain the understanding we need to make learning easier and more accessible to our children.

What Is Real?

As educators, we are constantly being made aware of the latest trends in education. Because no single approach can meet all needs, each new miracle cure is eventually found wanting, only to be replaced by yet another magic solution.

The truth is that there is no magic. Instead of being swayed now by one trend, now by another, we anchor our teaching in sound educational practice. We do this by approaching each situation from several angles.

- We hone our diagnostic skills. Our "explicit attempts to diagnose the content and articulateness of the child's [learning] schema" (Kagan 1968, 82) enable us to plan interventions that meet children's needs.
- We take our cues from children, offering them the skills and concepts they need as their interests and abilities develop.
- Insofar as possible, we include children in the process of defining problems and developing problem-solving strategies. We systematically analyze what has worked and what has not. This understanding informs our judgment as new situations present themselves.
- We examine our own experience, that of colleagues, and the findings of educational research. We draw on all of these, selecting what we need in order to develop in chil-

dren an awareness of their potential, along with the learning required to achieve it.

As we work, we forge the substance and style of our teaching by patience and perseverance, selecting and adapting, and by allowing ourselves to be influenced by our experience. It is our carefully considered experience, not fads or formulas, that enables us to respond wisely and effectively to the infinitely varied circumstances of resource room teaching.

Appendix A

Glossary of Terms

The following terms are found in *Profiles of Children* (see Appendix B).

Aided: With the use of hearing aids.

Conductive Loss: Hearing impairment due to failure of sound to be transmitted to the inner ear. Typical conductive hearing losses in children are caused by otitis media (middle ear infections), perforation of the tympanic membrane, and accumulation of wax in the external canal. In addition, congenital malformation of the ossicles (bones in the middle ear) can result in moderate to severe hearing losses. Many conductive conditions can be treated and hearing improved.

dBHL: Decibels Hearing Level

Frequency: Pitch.

Hertz (Hz): Frequency expressed in cycles per second.

Normal Conversational Level: 50 dBHL.

Sensorineural Loss: Permanent hearing impairment resulting from damage to the cochlea or auditory nerve.

Soundfield: Testing done in a soundproof room without headphones. Speakers are used to present sounds and words as they would normally be heard.

Speech Discrimination Ability: Percent of monosyllabic words a child can repeat accurately when presented by the audiologist at the child's most comfortable listening level; younger children identify pictures.

Speech Reception Threshold: Volume at which a child correctly repeats 50% of a phonetically balanced spondee word list (e.g., cupcake, baseball, mailman).

Symmetrical Loss: Same or nearly the same in both ears.

Unaided: Without the use of hearing aids.

Appendix B

Profiles of Children

The Audiologist's Report

The audiological information in the following profiles was gathered from evaluations by hospitals, clinics, and other testing facilities. Many of these reports contained a full range of hearing measurements. Several audiologists, when contacted, were able to supply essential information that had not been included in their original reports to the school. In other instances, information could not be supplied by the audiologists.

Teachers and children benefit when audiological reports include the following information.

- Immittance measurements (tympanograms) indicating middle ear status. Unlike sensorineural loss, which is essentially stable, conductive loss due to otitis media fluctuates according to the child's health. An abnormal tympanogram alerts the teacher to the effects of colds, congestion, or allergies on the child's hearing.
- The nature and extent of the child's hearing loss; the impact of the loss on the child's ability to hear speech in a quiet setting at close range, in contrast to the less than optimal classroom environment.
- A description of the child's ability to perceive speech with and without amplification. A comparison of these scores clarifies both the benefits and the limitations of the child's hearing aids and FM unit.
- An explanation of the audiologist's recommendations.

Audiologists enlighten teachers when they translate technical information derived from testing into verbal descriptions. A description that spells out the implications of a child's hearing loss with regard to classroom management, speech and language performance, classroom performance, and auditory training is more valuable to teachers than test results alone.

Belinda

- Unilateral sensorineural loss. Right ear severe, flat; left ear borderline normal. Wears no hearing aids.
- Unaided Speech Reception Threshold: 75 dBHL (right); 20 dBHL (left).
- Unaided Speech Discrimination at normal conversational level: 80% (right); 96% (left).

Belinda's kindergarten teacher was alerted to a possible hearing problem by the child's extreme inattention and difficulty focusing. A hearing loss was detected by a routine hearing screening and confirmed by further testing. A unilateral loss can have a significant impact on auditory and language development, but Belinda's parents have refused trial amplification. Belinda's lack of focus and difficulty in all academic areas have persisted throughout elementary school.

Cathy

- Bilateral conductive hearing loss. Right ear moderate, flat; left ear borderline mild to moderate, flat. Wears two hearing aids.
- Aided Speech Reception Threshold: 15 dBHL.
- Aided Speech Discrimination at normal conversational level: 96%; 92% at quiet level.

Hearing aids bring Cathy's hearing within the normal range. Nevertheless, Cathy experiences severe difficulties with the mechanics of reading, writing, and math. She displays similar deficits in all aspects of language and general knowledge. Cathy has difficulty following directions and discussions, even in her special education class for children with learning disabilities. Her deficits appear to be related to an auditory processing problem.

Crystal

- Bilateral sensorineural loss. Right ear mild sloping to moderate-severe at 500 Hz and to severe at 1000 Hz; left ear

severe sloping to profound. Wears hearing aid in right ear.
- Aided Speech Reception Threshold: 25 dBHL.
- Aided Speech Discrimination at 40 dB (her most comfortable listening level): 68% (right); no response (left).

Crystal experiences difficulty with speech discrimination even with amplification. Difficulties in spelling, math, and abstract concepts involving spatial relations suggest learning disabilities in addition to her hearing loss. Crystal evidences moderate language delays in vocabulary, grammar, and syntax. Nevertheless, she is a superior user of language, who by third grade revealed her grasp of nuances and ability to read with deep and active comprehension without necessarily understanding every word.

Curtis

- Bilateral symmetrical sensorineural loss. Mild to 750 Hz, sloping to moderate, and dropping to profound at 3000 Hz. Wears hearing aids inconsistently.
- Aided Speech Reception Threshold: 30 dBHL.
- Aided Speech Discrimination at normal conversational level: 68%.

Curtis entered the resource room program in second grade speaking no English. With no language reinforcement at home, his English was slow in developing. In spite of vocabulary deficits and grammatical and syntactical errors, Curtis has become a fairly competent language user. At age twelve, he expresses himself in simple and compound, but seldom complex sentences. A recent evaluation describes him as having above average analytic reasoning ability. Curtis is able to relate experiences and stories in a logical but brief manner. Curtis' mother has difficulty supporting the consistent use of hearing aids.

Cynthia

- Bilateral symmetrical sensorineural loss. Moderate-severe sloping to profound. Wears two hearing aids.
- Aided Speech Reception Threshold: 35 dBHL.
- Aided Speech Discrimination at normal conversational level: 68%.

Cynthia converses easily and appropriately in spite of her severe hearing loss. Her speech contains multiple articulation errors but can generally be understood without contextual clues.

At age twelve, she describes events in a well-related fashion, though with deficits in grammar and syntax: "When I hit the ball, then I would run to the first base." Irregular attendance has affected Cynthia's learning, in spite of her superior intelligence.

Dahlia

- Bilateral symmetrical sensorineural loss. Mild sloping to moderate-severe. Wears hearing aids inconsistently.
- Aided Speech Reception Threshold: 25 dBHL.
- Aided Speech Discrimination at normal conversational level: 100% (92% with background noise). Without hearing aids, Dahlia's discrimination drops to 68% at slightly softer than normal conversational level.

Dahlia's low language level in spite of considerable hearing reflects, in part, her limited exposure to English outside of school. In addition, Dahlia's mother has difficulty accepting her daughter's hearing loss and supporting the consistent use of hearing aids. Dahlia's hearing loss alone does not account for her difficulty with memory and abstract concepts.

Dominique

- Bilateral symmetrical conductive loss. Moderate rising to mild at 2000 Hz, dropping to moderate at 6000 Hz. Wears two hearing aids.
- Aided Speech Reception Threshold: 40 dBHL (right); 35 dBHL (left).
- Unaided Speech Discrimination at 65 dB: 92% (right); 96% (left).

Dominique has continued to experience extreme difficulty with auditory and visual perception as well as with concept development. Her verbal skills remain limited and concrete. After several years in regular classes, Dominique was placed in a self-contained class for children with learning disabilities.

Douglas

- Bilateral symmetrical sensorineural hearing loss. Moderate to severe through 500 Hz, sloping to severe. Wearing hearing aids since age five and one-half.
- Aided Speech Reception Threshold: 35 dBHL.
- Aided Speech Discrimination at normal conversational level: 72%.

With hearing aids, Douglas does well when close to the speaker in a quiet setting. Vocabulary, syntax, reading, and abstract thinking ability have developed remarkably since Douglas began wearing hearing aids. At age eight, however, Douglas continues to need individual support to understand stories fully or participate in discussions. He is just beginning to write stories in a one-to-one situation.

Emily

- Bilateral mild to moderate sensorineural loss. Wears two hearing aids.
- Unaided Speech Reception Threshold: 40 dBHL (right); 30 dBHL (left).
- Unaided Speech Discrimination: 80% (right at 75 dB); 72% (left at 65 dB).

Hearing aids bring Emily's hearing within normal limits. Her speech is free of articulation errors. Emily had a difficult early medical history related to prematurity and low birth weight. She displays difficulties suggestive of a learning disability. Emily is slow to acquire new vocabulary and language concepts. She has difficulty focusing, following a story line, and responding to basic questions.

Jerry

- Bilateral symmetrical sensorineural loss. Mild to 1000 Hz sloping sharply to severe at 4000 Hz. Wears hearing aids inconsistently.
- Aided Speech Reception Threshold: 15 dBHL.
- Aided Speech Discrimination at normal conversation level: 92% (80% with background noise).

Jerry speaks softly, with mild misarticulations. He avoids eye contact. Responses are concrete and limited in scope. At eight-and-one-half years of age, Jerry scored 3.7 in receptive vocabulary. At age twelve he had difficulty reading words such as "swallow" and "discover." Errors in opposites began at a basic level (asleep/outsleep, shut/unshut). Jerry recognized absurdities, but could explain what was wrong in fewer than half the statements. Inconsistent amplification due to parental ambivalence has exacerbated Jerry's difficulty in language learning.

Jimmy

- Bilateral sensorineural loss. Moderate to 500 Hz sloping to profound at 1000 Hz. Wears two hearing aids.
- Aided Speech Reception Threshold: 25 dBHL.
- Aided Speech Discrimination at normal conversational level: 48%.

Jimmy distorts many sounds and substitutes some sounds for others. He speaks in a relative monotone. Jimmy has received ongoing speech and language support services since preschool. In view of this, his language development appears slower than might be expected, even taking into account his substantial hearing loss.

John

- Bilateral symmetrical sensorineural loss. Mild to 2000 Hz sloping to severe at 8000 Hz. Wears two hearing aids fairly consistently.
- Aided Speech Reception Threshold: 20 dBHL.
- Aided Speech Discrimination at normal conversational level: 84% (right); 92% (left).

John's hearing loss went undiagnosed until age nine, when he began to wear hearing aids for the first time. At ten-and-one-half years of age, John scored in the first percentile in receptive language and auditory memory. His intellectual curiosity is, nevertheless, apparent as he ponders whether children outside of New York City could possibly be familiar with the Statue of Liberty: "I mean they never seen one or came to it, and they might not know how does it look or what does it called."

Joshua

- Bilateral symmetrical sensorineural hearing loss. Mild through 1000 Hz sloping to moderate. Wears two hearing aids.
- Aided Speech Discrimination at normal conversational level: 84% (right); 76% (left).

Joshua understands a good amount of speech through hearing alone in a quiet environment. With hearing aids, he hears comfortably at a normal conversational level. Joshua converses easily about the events of everyday life: "Douglas hit Robert." "You said I could take a book." Both auditory and visual memory are severely impaired, making it difficult for Joshua to acquire new words by listening or reading.

Nancy

- Bilateral sensorineural hearing loss. Right ear normal sharply sloping to profound at 1000 Hz; left ear severe to profound.
- Aided Speech Reception Threshold: 50 dBHL (right); 95 dBHL (left).
- Aided Speech Discrimination: Could not test due to lack of language.

At age six, Nancy has just begun to wear hearing aids and is receiving her first training in language development. Her articulation is severely delayed, resulting in poor intelligibility. Nancy is highly distractible. Her language level is that of a preverbal child: she mimics language, gestures, and facial expressions. Nancy can name and/or identify a handful of common objects. She has not yet learned to respond to "Who?" or "What?" questions.

Robert

- Bilateral symmetrical sensorineural hearing loss. Mild sloping to moderate.
- Unaided Speech Reception Threshold: 40 dBHL.
- Aided Speech Discrimination at normal conversational level: 96%.

Robert hears best when close to the speaker in a quiet setting. Without hearing aids, Robert's speech discrimination drops to 80%; background noise and distance from the speaker further reduce his ability to hear. Because of parental ambivalence regarding amplification, this situation frequently prevails. Robert uses the FM unit inconsistently in class, and wears no hearing aids outside of school. Robert has a well-developed language base, but with severe deficits in many areas.

Shelley

- Bilateral symmetrical sensorineural loss. Mild to 250 Hz sloping to moderate-severe through 1000 Hz and dropping sharply to profound at 1500 Hz. Wears hearing aid in right ear.
- Unaided Speech Reception Threshold: 65 dBHL (right); 55 dBHL (left).

- Aided Speech Discrimination at normal conversational level: 72% (64% at quiet level).

Shelley speaks in full, complex sentences, but with grammatical and syntactical errors. Formal testing reveals a paucity of vocabulary, and inadequate reasoning of the kind necessary for synonym/antonym formation and verbal analogies. Shelley converses fluently, with sibilant misarticulations and a somewhat flat intonation. Her intelligibility is fair at a simple phrase level, and decreases as phrase and sentence length increase.

Tom

- Bilateral symmetrical sensorineural loss. Mild sloping to moderate-severe at 1000 Hz and to severe at 1500 Hz. Wears two hearing aids.
- Aided Speech Reception Threshold: 45 dBHL.
- Aided Speech Discrimination at normal conversational level: 76% (40% at quiet level).

Tom's intelligibility is fair to poor, with many misarticulations. His low language and reading scores reflect, in part, his lack of exposure to English outside of school. Tom is an avid and purposeful learner who has developed strategies to supplement his hearing. He leans forward toward the speaker to listen. He indicates by the interrogative tone of his response when he is unsure of a question or statement. Tom repeats parts of previous sentences for confirmation, and requests repetition when necessary.

Bibliography of Children's Literature

Asch, Frank. 1984. *Moongame.* New York: Scholastic, Inc.

Baum, Frank L. 1988. *The Wizard of Oz.* Morris Plains, NJ: The Unicorn Publishing House, Inc.

Baylor, Byrd. 1989. *Amigo.* New York: Aladdin Books.

Berenstain, Stan. 1985. *The Berenstain Bears Learn About Strangers.* New York: Random House.

Bernos de Gasztold, Carmen. 1962. The Prayer of the Old Horse. In *Prayers from the Ark,* translated by Rumer Godden. New York: Viking Penquin.

Blishen, Edward, ed. 1963. Robin Hood and the Bishop of Hereford, This Is the Key, and Who Has Seen the Wind? In *Oxford Book of Poetry for Children.* Oxford: Oxford University Press.

Boning, Richard. 1976. *Specific Skills Series.* Baldwin, New York: Barnell Loft, Ltd.

Bridwell, Norman. 1963. *Clifford the Big Red Dog.* New York: Scholastic Book Services.

Brown, Margaret Wise. 1947. *Goodnight Moon.* New York: HarperCollins Publishers.

Bulla, Clyde Robert. 1987. *The Chalkbox Kid.* New York: Random House.

Catling, Patrick Skene. 1988. *The Chocolate Touch.* New York: Bantam Skylark.

Chisholm, Jane. 1982. *Living in Prehistoric Times.* London: Usborne Publishing Ltd.

Clymer, Eleanor. 1971. *The Spider, the Cave and the Pottery Bowl.* New York: Dell Publishing.

Cowley, Joy, and others. 1986. *Sunshine Core Programs.* Bothell, WA: The Wright Group.

Dalgliesh, Alice. 1954. *The Courage of Sarah Noble.* New York: Charles Scribner's Sons.

dePaola, Tomi. 1983. *The Legend of the Bluebonnet.* New York: G.P. Putnam's Sons.

Donnelly, Judy. 1987. *The Titanic: Lost . . . and Found.* New York: Random House.

Durr, William K. et al. 1983. Houghton Mifflin Reading Program. Boston: Houghton Mifflin Co.

Ferris, Jeri. 1988. *Go Free or Die: A Story About Harriet Tubman.* Minneapolis, MN: Carolrhoda Books, Inc.

Gallimard, Jeunesse, and Pierre Verdet. 1989. *The Earth and the Sky.* New York: Scholastic Inc.

Grimm, Brothers. 1980. *Hansel and Gretel.* New York: Dial Books for Young Children.

Hughes, Langston. 1994. City. In *Collected Poems.* New York: Alfred A. Knopf.

Hurley, William. 1966. *Dan Frontier.* Chicago, IL: Benefic Press.

Kaufman, John. 1982. *Bats in the Dark.* New York: Scholastic Book Services.

Krauss, Ruth. 1989. *The Carrot Seed.* New York: HarperCollins Publishers.

Krensky, Stephen. 1989. *It Happened in Salem Village.* New York: Random House.

Kumin, Maxine. 1986. *The Microscope.* New York: Harper Trophy.

Lepscky, Ibi. 1982. *Albert Einstein.* Hauppauge, New York: Barron's.

Lewis, Shari. 1990. *One-Minute Stories of Great Americans.* New York: Doubleday.

Liddle, William. 1977. *Reading for Concepts.* New York: Webster Division, McGraw-Hill Book Company.

Lindgren, Astrid. 1970. *Pippi Longstocking.* New York: Penguin Books U.S.A. Inc.

Lobel, Arnold. 1995. *Frog and Toad.* New York: HarperCollins Children's Books.

McCullagh, S. K. 1958. *Roderick the Red.* Leeds, England: E. J. Arnold and Son Ltd.

Merriam, Eve. 1984. A Lazy Thought. In *Jamboree Rhymes for All Times.* New York: Dell Yearling.

Munsch, Robert. 1985. *Mortimer.* Toronto: Annick Press Ltd.

Ogle, Lucille, and Thoburn, Tina. 1970. *I Spy.* New York: American Heritage Press.

Provensen, Alice and Martin. 1987. *The Glorious Flight.* New York: Viking Penguin.

Rawls, Wilson. 1974. *Where the Red Fern Grows.* New York: Bantam.

Riski, Maureen Cassidy, and Klakow, Nikolas. 1994. *Patrick Gets Hearing Aids.* Napierville, IL: Phonak Inc.

Roop, Jerry and Connie. 1985. *Keep the Lights Burning, Abbie.* Minneapolis, MN: Carolrhoda Books, Inc.

Roth, Susan. 1990. *Marco Polo: His Notebook.* New York: Doubleday.

Sachar, Louis. 1985. *Sideways Stories from Wayside School.* New York: Avon Books.

Sachs, Marilyn. 1971. *The Bears' House.* New York: Avon Books.

Schick, Eleanor. 1980. *Home Alone.* New York: Dial Press.

Schwartz, David. 1985. *How Much is a Million?* New York: Scholastic Inc.

Smallman, Clare. 1986. *Outside-In.* Hauppauge, New York: Barron's.

Warner, Gertrude Chandler. 1989. *The Boxcar Children.* New York: Scholastic Inc.

Webster, James. 1968. *Brown Beauty.* London: Ginn and Co. Ltd.

Webster, James. 1968. *Sally the Seagull.* London: Ginn and Co. Ltd.

White, E. B. 1952. *Charlotte's Web.* New York: HarperCollins Publishers.

White, E. B. 1970. *Trumpet of the Swan.* New York: HarperCollins Publishers.

Wilder, Laura Ingalls. 1953. *Little House on the Prairie.* New York: HarperCollins Publishers.

Williams, Vera B. 1982. *A Chair for My Mother.* New York: Greenwillow Books.

Wilson, Jean. 1974. *Children of Ancient Greece.* Reading, MA: Addison-Wesley Publishing Co.

Yashima, Taro. 1976. *Crow Boy.* New York: Puffin Books.

Ziefert, Harriet. 1988. *Mommy, Where Are You?* New York: Viking Penguin.

Zolotow, Charlotte. 1985. *William's Doll.* New York: HarperCollins Publishers.

Works Cited

Adams, Marilyn J. 1991. Why not Phonics and Whole Language? In *All Language and the Creation of Literacy*, edited by William Ellis. Baltimore, MD: Orton Dyslexia Society.

Adams, Marilyn J., and Bruck, Maggie. 1995. Resolving the Great Debate. *American Educator* 19, 2 (Summer): 7, 10–19.

Adams, Marilyn J., and Bruck, Maggie. 1993. Word Recognition: The Interface of Educational Policies and Scientific Research. *Reading and Writing: An Interdisciplinary Journal* 5: 113–39.

Anderson, Karen L., and Matkin, Noel D. 1991. Relationship of Degree of Long Term Hearing Loss to Psychosocial and Educational Needs. Adapted from *Relationship of Hearing Impairment to Educational Needs* (Bernero and Bothwell 1966). Illinois Department of Public Health and Office of Superintendent of Public Instruction.

Anderson, Richard, and Nagy, William. 1992. The Vocabulary Conundrum. *American Educator* (Winter): 14-18, 44–47.

Anderson, Richard C., Hiebert, Elfrieda H., Scott, Judith A., and Wilkinson, Ian A.G. 1985. *Becoming a Nation of Readers*. Washington, DC: The National Institute of Education.

Ashton-Warner, Sylvia. 1963. *Teacher*. New York: Simon and Schuster.

Avery, Carol. 1993. *". . . And with a Light Touch"*. Portsmouth, NH: Heinemann.

Axline, Virginia M. 1964. *Dibs in Search of Self*. New York: Ballantine Books, Inc.

Beck, Isabel L., and Juel, Connie. 1995. The Role of Decoding in Learning to Read. In *American Educator* 19, 2 (Summer): 8, 21–25, 39–42.

Beck, Isabel L., McKeown, Margaret G., and McCaslin, Ellen S. 1981. Does Reading Make Sense? Problems of Early Readers. *The Reading Teacher* 34: 780–85.

Beebe, Helen Hulick. 1953. *A Guide to Help the Severely Hard of Hearing Child*. New York: S. Karger.

Bell, Nanci. 1986. *Visualizing and Verbalizing*. Paso Robles, CA: Academy of Reading Publications.

Bess, Fred H., Freeman, Barry A., and Sinclair, J. Stephen, eds. 1981. *Amplification in Education*. Washington, DC: The Alexander Graham Bell Society for the Deaf.

Bettelheim, Bruno. 1989. *The Uses of Enchantment: The Meaning and Importance of Fairy Tales*. New York: Random House, Inc.

Birch, Jack W. 1975. *Hearing-Impaired Children in the Mainstream.* Minneapolis, MN: U.S. Office of Education.

Bloom, Benjamin S. 1984. The 2 Sigma Problem: The Search for Methods of Group Instruction as Effective as One-to-One Tutoring. *Educational Research* 13, 6 (June-July): 4–16.

Bloom, Lois. 1995. Forward. See Hart, Betty, and Risley, Todd R.

Boothroyd, Arthur. 1988. *Hearing Impairments in Young Children.* Washington, DC: The Alexander Graham Bell Association for the Deaf.

Brackett, Diane. 1990. Communication of Mainstreamed Hearing-Impaired Students. *Hearing-Impaired Children in the Mainstream,* ed. Mark Ross. Timonium, MD: York Press.

Bransford, J.D., Stein, Barry S., Vye, Nancy J., Franks, Jeffrey J., Auble, Pamela M., Mezynski, Karen J., and Perfetto, Greg A. 1982. Differences in Approaches to Learning: An Overview. *Journal of Experimental Psychology: General.* 111: 390–98.

Breene, Michael, and Candlin, Christopher. 1980. Essentials of a Communication Curriculum. *Applied Linguistics* 1, 2 (Summer): 89–112

Bruner, Jerome. 1983. *Child's Talk: Learning to Use Language.* New York: W. W. Norton and Company.

Bruner, Jerome. 1978. The Role of Dialogue in Language Acquisition. In *The Child's Conception of Language,* eds. A. Sinclair and others. New York: Springer Verlag.

Butler, Dorothy, and Clay, Marie. 1979. *Reading Begins at Home.* Portsmouth, NH: Heinemann Educational Books.

Calkins, Lucy McCormick. 1983. *Lessons From A Child: On the Teaching and Learning of Writing.* Portsmouth, NH: Heinemann Educational Books.

Calkins, Lucy McCormick with Harwayne, Shelley. 1991. *Living Between the Lines.* Portsmouth, NH: Heinemann Educational Books.

Capper, Colleen. 1989. *Transformative Leadership: Embracing Student Diversity in Democratic Schooling* (January): ERIC ED 305 714.

Carbo, Marie. 1987. Deprogramming Reading Failure: Giving Unequal Learners an Equal Chance. *Phi Delta Kappan* 69, 3 (November): 197–202.

Carbo, Marie. 1997. *What Every Principal Should Know About Teaching Reading.* Syosset, New York: National Reading Styles Institute.

Casanave, Suki. 1991. A Community of Friends and Classmates. *Equity and Choice* 8, 1 (Fall): 38–44.

Center for Assessment and Demographic Studies. 1991. *Stanford Achievement Test (8th Edition, Form J): Hearing Impaired Norms Booklet.* Washington, DC: Gallaudet Research Institute (February).

Chall, Jean. 1967. *Learning to Read: The Great Debate.* New York: McGraw-Hill, Inc.

Code of Federal Regulations (CFR): Title 34; Education; Parts 1 to 399 (July 1, 1993). Washington, DC: U.S. Government Printing Office.

Cutting, Brian. [1990.] *Getting Started in Whole Language.* Bothell, WA: The Wright Group.

de Maupassant, Guy. 1967. The Necklace. In *Favorite Short Stories,* ed. Lewis G. Sterner. New York: Globe Book Company.

Donaldson, Margaret. 1978. *Children's Minds.* New York: W.W. Norton.

Ellis, Rod. 1985. Teacher-pupil Interaction in Second Language Development. In *Input in Second Language Acquisition,* eds. Susan M. Gass and Carolyn G. Madden. Rowley, MA: Newbury House.

Fader, Daniel with Duggins, James, Finn, Tom, and McNeil, Elton. 1976. *The New Hooked On Books.* New York: Berkley Publishing Corp.

Fernald, Grace. 1943. *Remedial Techniques in Basic School Subjects.* New York: McGraw-Hill Book Co., Inc.

Flesch, Rudolf Franz. 1955. *Why Johnny Can't Read.* New York: HarperCollins Publishers.

Foran, Katherine, and Heim, David. 1994. Helping Your Child Succeed in School. *Adoptive Families* (September-October): 22–24.

Foster, Susan. 1989. Reflections of a Group of Deaf Adults on their Experiences in Mainstream and Residential School Programs in the United States. In *Disability, Handicap and Society* 4,1: 55.

Freeman, Mary Wilkins. 1967. The Revolt of Mother. In *Favorite Short Stories*, ed. Lewis G. Sterner. New York: Globe Book Company.

Gillingham, Anna, and Stillman, Bessie W. 1965. *Remedial Training for Children with Specific Disability in Reading, Spelling and Penmanship.* Cambridge, MA: Educators Publishing Services, Inc.

Graves, Donald H. 1989. *Investigate Non-Fiction.* Portsmouth, NH: Heinemann.

Griffing, Barry L. 1970. Planning Educational Programs and services for Hard of Hearing Children. In *The Hard of Hearing Child: Clinical and Educational Management*, eds. Frederick S. Berger and Samuel G. Fletcher. New York: Grune and Stratton.

Haley, Gail. 1975. In *Newbery and Caldecott Medal Books 1966–1975*, ed. Lee Kingman. Boston: Horn Book.

Hart, Archibald. 1964. *Twelve Ways to Build a Vocabulary.* New York: Barnes and Noble.

Hart, Betty, and Risley, Todd R. 1995. *Meaningful Differences in the Everyday Experiences of Young American Children.* Baltimore, MD: Paul H. Brookes Publishing Co.

Horowitz, Frances Degen. 1995. *Human Potential at Risk—Environmental Contexts.* Paper presented at American Psychological Association Annual Meeting. New York City.

Huefner, Dixie Snow. 1988. The Consulting Teacher Model: Risks and Opportunities. *Exceptional Children* 54, 5: 403–14.

Jenkins, Joseph R., and Jenkins, Linda M. 1981. *Cross-Age and Peer Tutoring: Help for Children with Learning Problems.* Reston, VA: Council for Exceptional Children.

Johnson, David W., Johnson, Roger T., Holubec, Edythe Johnson, and Roy, Patricia. 1984. *Circles of Learning: Cooperation in the Classroom.* Minneapolis, MN: Association for Supervision and Curriculum Development.

Just, M.A., and Carpenter, P.A. 1987. *The Psychology of Reading and Language Comprehension.* Boston: Allyn and Bacon.

Kagan, Jerome. 1968. The Child: His Struggle for Identity. *Saturday Review* 51, 49 (7 December): 80–82, 87–88.

Katz, Lilian. 1993. "All About Me": Are We Developing Our Children's Self-Esteem or their Narcissism? *American Educator* (Summer): 18–23.

Kirchner, Carl. 1995. The Inclusive Environment. *Hearing Health* 11, 5 (September-October): 37, 38–40.

Krashen, Stephen. 1982. Providing Input for Acquisition. In *Principles and Practice in Second Language Acquisition.* Oxford: Pergamon.

Lerner, Barbara. 1996. Self-Esteem and Excellence: The Choice and the Paradox. In *American Educator* 20, 2 (Summer): 9–13, 41.

Levine, Melvin. 1994. *Educational Care.* Cambridge, MA: Educators Publishing Service, Inc.

Limbrick, E.A., McNaughton, S., and Clay, Marie. 1992. Time Engaged in Reading: A Critical Factor in Reading Achievement. *American Annals of the Deaf* 137, 4 (October): 309–14.

Macdonald, Cathy, and York, Jennifer. 1989. Instruction in Regular Education Classes for Students with Severe Disabilities: Assessment, Objectives, and Instructional Programs. *Strategies for Full Inclusion.* ERIC ED. 338 638.

Meyers, Joel, Gelzheiser, Lynn M., and Yelich, Glen. 1991. Do Pull-In Programs Foster Teacher Collaboration? *Remedial and Special Education* 12, 2 (March-April): 7–15.

Miller, Kevin, and Luckner, John. 1992. Let's Talk About It: Using Conversation to Facilitate Language Development. *American Annals of the Deaf* 137, 4 (October): 345–50.

Mueller, H. Gustav, Hawkins, David B., and. Northern, Jerry L. 1992. *Probe Microphone Measurements: Hearing Aid Selection and Assessment.* San Diego, CA: Singular.

Murphy, Lois Barclay, and Hirschberg, J. Cotter. 1982. *Robin: Comprehensive Treatment of a Vulnerable Adolescent.* New York: Basic Books.

Norris, Janet A., and Damico, Jack S. 1990. Whole Language in Theory and Practice: Implications for Language Intervention. *Language, Speech, and Hearing in Schools* 21, 4 (October): 212–220.

O'Connor, Johnson. 1964. Preface to *Twelve Ways to Build A Vocabulary.* See Hart, Archibald.

Oller, John W., Jr. 1983. Some Working Ideas for Language Teaching. In *Methods That Work: A Smorgasbord of Ideas for Language Teachers,* eds. J. Oller, Jr. and Patricia Richard-Amato. Rowley, MA: Newbery House.

Patrizio, Alexis. 1995. A Graduate Speaks. *The Listening Post* (Spring): 4–5. (Available from The Helen Beebe Center, 220 Commerce Drive, Suite 302, Fort Washington, PA 19034).

Piaget, Jean. 1968. *Judgment and Reasoning in the Child.* Totowa, NJ: Littlefield, Adams and Co.

Reisberg, Lenny, and Wolf, Ronald. 1986. Developing a Consulting Program in Special Education: Implementation and Intervention. *Focus on Exceptional Children* 19, 3 (November): 1–14.

Richard-Amato, Patricia. 1996. *Making It Happen: Interaction in the Second Language Classroom.* White Plains, NY: Longman.

Robinson, Kathy. 1987. *Children of Silence: The Story of My Daughters' Triumph Over Deafness.* New York: E.P. Dutton.

Ross, Mark, Brackett, Diane, and Maxon, Antonia Brancia. 1991. *Assessment and Management of Mainstreamed Hearing-Impaired Children.* Austin, TX: PRO-ED, Inc.

Sheirer, John. 1993. I Think, Therefore I Question. *NewsSmith* (Summer): 12. (Available from Smith College, Northhampton, MA 01063).

Smith, Frank. 1985. *Reading Without Nonsense.* New York: Teachers College Press.

Snow, Catherine E., and Ninio, Anat. 1986. The Contracts of Literacy: What Children Learn from Learning to Read Books. In *Emergent Literacy: Writing and Reading,* eds. William H. Teale and Elizabeth Sulzby. Norwood, NJ: Ablex Publishing Co.

Stanovich, K.E. 1986. Matthew Effect in Reading: Some Consequences of Individual Differences in the Acquisition of Literacy. *Reading Research Quarterly* 21, 4 (Fall): 360–407.

Stein, Nancy L., and Trabasso, Tom. 1982. What's in a Story? In *Advances in Instructional Psychology,* 2: 213–67, ed. Robert Glaser. Hillsdale, NJ: Lawrence Erlbaum Associates.

Swain, Merrill. 1985. Communication Competence: Some Roles of Comprehensible Input and Comprehensible Output In Its Development. In *Input in Se-*

cond Language Acquisition, eds. Susan M. Gass and Carolyn G. Madden. Rowley, MA: Newbury House.

Trelease, Jim. 1985. *The Read-Aloud Handbook*. New York: Penguin.

Truitt, Anne. 1984. *Daybook: The Journal of an Artist*. New York: Viking Penguin.

Vellutino, Frank R. 1991. Introduction to Three Studies on Reading Acquisition: Convergent Findings on Theoretical Foundations of Code-Oriented Versus Whole-Language Approaches to Reading Instruction. *Journal of Educational Psychology* 83, 4: 437–443.

Vygotsky, Lev. 1962. *Thought and Language*, trans. Eugenia Hanfmann et al. Cambridge, MA: MIT Press.

Winn, Marie. 1985. *The Plug-In Drug*. New York: Penguin Books.

York, Jennifer, and Vandercook, Terri. 1989. Strategies for Achieving an Integrated Education for Middle School Learners with Severe Disabilities. *Strategies for Full Inclusion*. ERIC ED 338 638.

Index